# Child Psychiatry and
# Child Protection Litigation

This study, one of four about expert evidence, was funded by the Department of Health and supported by the Lord Chancellor's Department; the views expressed, however, are those of the authors and not necessarily those of either Department.

JULIA BROPHY
with
LOUISE BROWN, SUZANNE COHEN
and POLLY RADCLIFFE

# Child Psychiatry and
# Child Protection Litigation

GASKELL

Gaskell is an imprint of the Royal College of Psychiatrists
17 Belgrave Square, London SW1X 8PG

**British Library Cataloguing-in-Publication Data**
A catalogue record for this book is available from
the British Library.
ISBN 1-901242-66-8

Distributed in North America
by American Psychiatric Press, Inc.

Printed in Great Britain by Bell & Bain Limited, Glasgow

For Carole, and Elizabeth

# Contents

# List of tables, boxes and figures

**Figure**

# Foreword

Perhaps the profoundest advance in the family justice system over the past decade has been the judicial recognition that good results depend upon interdisciplinary collaboration. The bond between the judge and any expert concerned with child health and development is particularly close since in some degree they share the daunting task of deciding the future of the child. The specialist judiciary owes a great debt to child psychiatry, whose consultants have, over the past decade, undertaken forensic work unstintingly, despite its rigours and frustrations. We, the judges, must neither take this service for granted nor assume that it will be as freely available in the future as it has been in the past.

Recognising this reality, the President's Interdisciplinary Committee has recently made a special commitment to the investigation of obstacles to the development of the forensic service and to planning for its future. This work is being done in collaboration with the Department of Health and the Lord Chancellor's Department.

However, there can be no doubt that it is the research of Julia Brophy that has galvanised the President's Interdisciplinary Committee into action. Her penetrative investigations and boldly stated conclusions have destroyed the complacency that can flourish in ignorance and they prove the need both to improve existing services and to lay the foundations for a better future.

The policy options posed by Julia are controversial and further exploration of the views and experiences of the child psychiatrists in this study would be important. Julia's writing invariably stimulates reflection and provokes debate – that is the purpose of good research. In the field she examines there is no room for indifference. I hope therefore that this admirable publication will be widely read and the issues that it raises debated, both formally and informally, among the membership of the Royal College of Psychiatrists. The future of the psychiatric contribution to the forensic process depends upon an awareness of the current problems and a commitment to their solution.

*The Rt Hon Lord Justice Thorpe*
*May 2001*

# Preface

The study on which this book is based is drawn from one of four interrelated studies about the use of experts in child protection litigation. Thus, the issues that it explores are drawn from findings from three previous linked studies designed to explore care proceedings following the Children Act 1989. The first of these (Bates & Brophy, 1996) was a court-based prospective study of care proceedings emanating from one local authority in England. This study tracked all new cases over a specified period utilising both qualitative and quantitative methods; the sample size was 65 cases concerning 114 children.

The second study in the project was a national random survey of guardians and of care and related proceedings. This national survey (Brophy *et al*, 1999*b*) explored a wide range of issues concerning the use of experts since the Act, including views about the use and availability of child and family mental health services for medico-legal purposes. In addition, the survey analysed 557 cases, concerning just under 1000 children, that contained expert evidence.

The penultimate study in the project focused on the work and decision-making of the guardian ad litem in complex cases involving expert evidence (Brophy & Bates, 1998, 1999). In this study, guardians were randomly selected from panels in three geographically diverse areas in England. In-depth semi-structured interviews were undertaken with 35 guardians exploring a range of issues about training, policy and practice regarding the use and work of experts. In addition, a complex decision-making exercise (based on a hypothetical case involving evidence from child psychiatrists) was undertaken with guardians.

Findings from these three studies raised a range of issues about current practices. Perhaps not least of these was the fact that, although a number of child welfare specialists (e.g. paediatricians, paediatric radiologists, adult psychiatrists, clinical and educational psychologists) might be instructed to provide assessments and reports for courts, nationally child and adolescent psychiatrists were identified as the major providers of expert evidence. Findings from the first three studies raised various issues and concerns about practices following the Children Act 1989. However, what was missing at that time were the views and experiences of child psychiatrists –those on the receiving end of a new legal agenda – who, nevertheless, remained willing to undertake this work. These views, practices and experiences were therefore pursued in in-depth interviews with a selected sample of 17 such specialists, and that study provides the data on which this book is based. The criteria for the selection of child psychiatrists and the full methodology are outlined in the Appendix. All interviews were taped and fully transcribed.

Family policy and family law seldom stand still and that is especially the case in the field of child protection litigation. During the period between completion of the study and its release for publication there have been a number of changes, many of which have implications for practices in the field we have explored.

As this study illustrates, the family justice system is heavily dependent on contributions from a number of agencies (social services, legal and health services) and a range of professionals (social workers, lawyers, guardians, magistrates, court clerks and judges, and child welfare specialists across a range of disciplines). Thus, changes to policies outside of legal proceedings can have a significant effect on attitudes towards and practices within the legal arena. This study has seen a range of changes during its gestation, not least of which was a change of government in the UK. Policy initiatives following that change, in law, social services and the National Health Service (NHS) have, or will probably have, implications for almost all the professionals likely to be involved in public law proceedings concerning allegations of child maltreatment by parents.

Where possible these subsequent changes or their possible implications have been highlighted in the text as areas that require careful monitoring and further research. So, for example, in the immediate field explored in this study (Child and Adolescent Mental Health Services) changes within the NHS such as reforms to the purchaser–provider split in health care and proposed changes to doctors' contracts, although not aimed at the provision of medico-legal services as such, are nevertheless likely to have an effect on medico-legal practices.

Equally, after the completion of this study the introduction of systems of 'mentoring' to enable willing specialist registrars to gain some experience in the legal arena should improve the supply of appropriately trained and experienced experts for the 'family justice system'.

In the field of social services, following this study a new framework was issued for social workers undertaking assessments of families, and the Quality Protects Programme aimed to transform the management and delivery of children's social services. With regard to court welfare services, in the spring of 2001 a single unified court welfare service (the Children and Families Courts Advice and Support Service (CAFCASS)) replaced two previous services (the Court Welfare Service and the Guardian ad Litem and Reporting Officers Service). Moreover, a new version of *Working Together* aimed to improve inter-agency cooperation between, for example, health and social services, and this in particular requires careful monitoring.

The introduction of a Legal Services Commission and the replacement of the Legal Aid Board with the Community Legal Service (CLS) Fund, together with the introduction of fixed fees for both lawyers and, in all probability, guardians working in this field may have an impact on the quality and availability of child welfare and legal specialists in this highly complex area. It would, for example, be a great loss to the family justice system if the most experienced practitioners ultimately withdrew from this type of work. As this study indicates, the quality of letters of instruction to child psychiatrists is an important component in decisions about whether they take on this type of work.

All these initiatives have implications for the policy field explored in this study. We have tried to demonstrate in the text where these issues might affect the views and experiences identified by specialists. What is without doubt is that for the above new initiatives to have a significant impact on improving the availability, quality and experiences of expert witnesses, the views and experiences of the child psychiatrists in this study should be addressed. For their agreement to participate in the study, for their patience, time, good humour and candid responses in this controversial field, we remain most grateful.

*Julia Brophy*
*Oxford Centre for Family Law and Policy*
*University of Oxford*

# Acknowledgements

This study was funded by the Department of Health and supported by the Lord Chancellor's Department. Thanks are due to the Advisory Committee: Carolyn Davies (Senior Principal Research Officer) and Arran Poyser (Social Services Inspector), Department of Health; Katherine Gieve (Solicitor, Bindman and Partners, London); Susan Golombok (Director, Clinical and Health Psychology Research Unit, City University); Eva Gregory (National Association of Guardians ad Litem and Reporting Officers); Jean Harris Hendriks (Consultant in Child and Adolescent Psychiatry); Mavis Maclean (Senior Research Fellow, Centre for Socio-Legal Studies, Wolfson College, Oxford); Panna Modi (Guardian ad Litem and Reporting Officer for the Leicester Panel, Consultant to the Nottingham Panel and Independent Assessor for the Birmingham Panel and Project Manager – Child Care, at the National Society for the Prevention of Cruelty to Children, Leicester); Neville Paul (Family Policy Division, Lord Chancellor's Department); and Mary Ryan (Co-Director, Family Rights Group). Particular thanks are due to the Chair of this Committee, Joyce Plotnikoff (Guardian ad Litem and independent consultant in civil and criminal justice).

Findings were presented at two closed seminars: Protecting Children, at the Centre for Socio-Legal Studies, Wolfson College, Oxford, and a meeting of the President's Interdisciplinary Family Law Committee. Thanks are due to colleagues at both meetings for their views and comments.

Many people showed an interest in this study and thanks for discussions and comments on an initial research report are due to: Carol Edwards (Appraiser and Trainer for the GALRO Service), Peter Hay (Area Manager, Social Services Department, Humberside County Council), Jane Hoyal (Barrister), Adrian James (Department of Applied Social Studies, University of Bradford), David Jones (Consultant Child and Adolescent Psychiatrist, Park Hospital for Children, Oxford), Judith Masson (School of Law, University of

Warwick), June Thoburn (School of Social Work, University of East Anglia) and Guinevere Tufnell (Consultant Child and Adolescent Psychiatrist, Thorpe Combe Hospital, London).

The study was based at the Thomas Coram Research Unit, Institute of Education, University of London, and thanks are due to colleagues in the Unit. Louise Brown, Suzanne Cohen and Polly Radcliffe were the research officers for this study and undertook some excellent work. Vivienne Metliss was the project administrator and I am indebted to her for her unstinting and professional work.

In addition to support from the Royal College of Psychiatrists, publication of this book is supported by a grant from the Nuffield Foundation and from the National Association of Guardians ad Litem and Reporting Officers (NAGALRO). Special thanks are due to Sharon Witherspoon, Assistant Director Social Research and Innovation at Nuffield, and to Susan Bindman (chair) and the Council of NAGALRO.

I would also like to thank Dr Caroline Lindsey, and Professor David Cottrell for very helpful suggestions and additional information regarding changes to training for specialist registrars following the completion of the study. For editorial support particular thanks go to Sheila Mellor. Any errors of course remain entirely my responsibility.

Finally, my thanks to the Rt Hon Lord Justice Thorpe for his support for the Expert Evidence Project as a whole and for writing the Foreword to this book.

Julia Brophy

# Introduction

Research demonstrates that although a range of medical and mental health specialists may be instructed in public law proceedings, following the enactment of the 1989 Children Act, child psychiatrists[1] are the major group of specialists providing assessments and reports for courts. Nationally, they are more likely to be instructed than are members of other professions, such as psychologists and adult psychiatrists, and they are the main specialists instructed by the professional parties in proceedings, that is, the local authority and the guardian ad litem (Brophy *et al*, 1999*b*, table 4.9), and this pattern applies to all children, regardless of ethnic group (Brophy, 2000*a*).

The study reported in this book is based on findings from in-depth interviews with a sample of 17 child psychiatrists[2] undertaken in 1996.[3] It focuses on their views and experiences of providing expert evidence in public law proceedings following the 1989 Children Act. In the UK, as in some other countries, there are comparatively few child psychiatrists relative to need,[4] and even fewer who are willing to

---

[1] The term child psychiatrist is used throughout this book, but this is not to imply a distinction from a child and adolescent psychiatrist.

[2] The sampling procedure is described in the Appendix. One of the selected psychiatrists was not in fact a child psychiatrist; however, because this consultant had a particular clinical and research interest in issues central to Children Act proceedings and had provided expert evidence in such cases, it was decided to retain this respondent in the sample.

[3] As indicated in the Preface, this study is one of four interrelated studies on expert evidence funded by the Department of Health and supported by the Lord Chancellor's Department. Other publications from the studies are listed in the references.

[4] For example, at May 2000, there were some 628 child and adolescent psychiatrists registered with the Royal College of Psychiatrists. No reliable information exists on the number who are able and willing to undertake instructions in public law proceedings, but indications suggest it is a very small proportion. For example, at the time of the fieldwork for this study, 19 clinicians were registered in the *Directory of Expert Witnesses* published by the Law Society (1996).

undertake instructions in public law proceedings. The aim of this study, therefore, was to provide very detailed information from a somewhat specialised subgroup of clinicians within child psychiatry as a whole – in sampling terms, what Patton (1990) calls the 'extreme or deviant case'. And as this study indicates, those child psychiatrists who do currently undertake this work may deviate in a number of important respects from mainstream child psychiatrists.

## *Background*

Before the Children Act 1989, there was very little empirical information on the use of experts in care proceedings.[5] None the less, the use of experts in the legal arena generally remained a controversial area (e.g. Smith & Wynne, 1989) and this is particularly the case with regard to psychological and psychiatric evidence (King, 1981; Lloyd-Bostock, 1981; King & Piper, 1990; Dent & Flin, 1992). Professional and academic debate about the use and impact of expert opinion was intensified not only by child abuse inquiries such as the Cleveland inquiry and report (Department of Health and Social Security, 1988) but also by pressure groups on behalf of parents such as the Family Rights Group and Parents Against Injustice. These developments increased awareness of the number and extent of clinical examinations to which children might be subject. But controversy in this field was not limited to clinical methods and the validity of interpretations made by experts in paediatrics and psychology or psychiatry.

At the heart of one debate generated by clinicians and academics are questions about the nature of expert knowledge in the field of child health and development and its application to legal questions. It has, for example, been argued that 'child welfare' and the 'law' adopt different methods, and this has particular implications for the way in which certain types of knowledge about children's welfare and development is being 'accommodated' in the legal arena. Before any research had been undertaken on proceedings under the Children Act, it was argued that these two disciplines and their attendant discourses and methodologies were inherently incompatible and, in the final analysis, legal methods and discourses, driven by notions of 'truth' and 'facts', dominate practices. In other words, 'law', by its very

---

[5] A few small-scale studies identified some limited use of experts in care proceedings before the 1989 Children Act (e.g. Coyle, 1985) but these did little beyond identifying that some experts had been instructed in cases (cf. Hunt, 1993; Plotnikoff & Wolfson, 1994).

nature, dominates and transforms child welfare knowledge, usually to the detriment of children (King, 1990; King & Piper, 1990; King & Trowell, 1992; cf. James, 1992).

After the Children Act, however, the debate about the lack of compatibility between the two discourses and methodologies was somewhat marginalised by two concerns, one about increased delay and costs in care proceedings since the Act, the other focusing on the overuse or inappropriate use of experts (e.g. Booth, 1996). In this latter respect it has, for example, been argued by child welfare specialists that limited resources in child health would be better aimed at therapeutic or preventive work with families, rather than invested in attempts at a forensic resolution of disputes between parents and local authorities (e.g. Spicer, 1996).

In addition, questions continued to arise about the degree to which experts act as hired guns for instructing parties, to rubber stamp decisions for local authorities or to do assessments that could or should have been undertaken by social workers. Equally, concern has been expressed about the degree to which experts attempt to make decisions that are the province of the judge. And broader debates about what constitutes 'hard' and 'soft' evidence continued (e.g. Betts, 1988; Gibson, 1988; Lyon, 1988; cf. Blom Cooper, 1988).

In courtroom practices, a quest for certainty in evidence from experts finds expression in what is termed the 'adversarial approach'. Here, advocates are said to continue to identify and take advantage of uncertainty in the evidence of the expert witness, or at least to gain an acknowledgement from an expert that an alternative interpretation and therefore opinion of a given situation is possible. Indeed, discrediting experts in the 'psy' professions has often been seen as fair and easy game for new advocates wishing to develop their advocacy skills (e.g. Napley, 1975; Evans, 1983; Hyam, 1992). For some child welfare specialists, experiences of being cross-examined by such advocates have led to a dislike and a refusal to enter the legal arena (see Lloyd-Bostock, 1988; King, 1991; Brophy *et al*, 1999*b*). That refusal has fuelled the debate about the incompatibility of the different methods and the continued domination of child welfare issues by the quest of the 'law' for certainty and truth.[6]

Despite those debates, during the late 1980s and throughout the 1990s dialogue between clinicians and lawyers, judges and academics

---

[6] It could also be the case that this debate has heightened inter-agency tensions and disputes between, for example, the local authority and child and family mental health services, although arguably inter-agency cooperation is likely to be at least equally affected by limited resources in CAMHS for forensic work.

continued to reassess and restructure what 'law' could expect from child welfare specialists (e.g. Carson, 1988; Wolkind, 1988; Golombok & Tasker, 1991; Brophy, 1992; Bull, 1992). Conversely, developments in case law and practice directions following the Children Act 1989 demonstrated that 'law' and legal procedures were engaged in a radical reshaping of the structure and processes through which expert knowledge reaches the legal arena. For some clinicians, changes introduced by the Children Act 1989 have been a source of disappointment and substantial criticism (e.g. Wolkind, 1993).[7] Legal practitioners (e.g. White, 1993), however, have argued that the disappointment experienced by clinicians is the fault of interpretation of the Act and a lack of resources, rather than a result of the legislation itself. In effect, it seems that in the new legislation we have a Rolls-Royce – but we can't afford to get it out of the garage. Despite the lack of resources, a number of revisions to legal procedure and substantive law have dramatically changed the agenda under which clinicians now bring child welfare knowledge to bear on the questions set by law in care proceedings. This study aimed to explore the views and experiences of a sample of child psychiatrists working at the interface of law and child welfare knowledge some five years after the implementation of a new, more child-centred public law regime.

## The sample

Research indicated considerable complexity in the avenues through which child psychiatrists are identified and instructed. In the early days of the Act at least, the evidence suggested that, in certain areas, the major parties (i.e. the local authority, the parents and the guardian ad litem) tended to draw on different pools of experts (Brophy & Bates, 1998). Thus, some experts routinely accepted instructions from parents, some from guardians and others from local authorities.

A full description of the sampling procedure is outlined in the Appendix. In brief, the study adopted a purposive sampling method (i.e. there were stated inclusion criteria), to obtain a sample of child psychiatrists that included clinicians from a range of these pools of experts identified above, and from both 'local' child and adolescent mental health services (CAMHS) and from a national network from which all parties might also draw. In certain respects, the distinctions

---

[7] Wolkind (1993, pp. 40–41) argued that "after one year's experience of the Act it seemed that this was written by lawyers and civil servants with remarkably little idea about the realities of disturbed children and of complex family dynamics".

between local and national proved to be more ideal types than distinct and unrelated groups. Some of the issues examined during interviews indicated some overlap between these two categories.[8] However, the categories were maintained, partly because they provided a useful framework for describing the institutional/employment basis of consultants, and partly because there were some important features of practice (e.g. the likelihood of clinical involvement with families before proceedings and the ability to offer treatment for children once proceedings were concluded) that were specific to each category.

Chapter 2 characterises the sample further. Quotations are attributed to individual experts designated by L for 'local' or N for 'national' and sample number.

## The structure of the book

Chapter 1 outlines the aims, objectives and specific provisions of the Children Act 1989 as these relate to public law proceedings, along with the duties and responsibilities of experts as these have been and continue to be developed by practice directions, case law and research findings. Chapter 1 also outlines trends in the use of experts in care proceedings from all disciplines since the introduction of the Children Act 1989.

Chapter 2 examines the employment/contractual context in which child psychiatrists generally undertake this type of medico-legal work – the context in which they provide a service for courts *and* parties. This chapter also explores how the contractual context influences the referrals experts are likely to accept, the services they can generally offer and the resources and ethical issues that certain referrals raise.

Research demonstrates that public law proceedings under the Children Act are characterised by a relatively high use of expertise beyond that of social workers and guardians. Thus, Chapter 3 examines the range of questions routinely put to child psychiatrists, perceptions of their 'added value' to cases and the techniques and underlying theoretical perspectives on which they draw. This chapter also explores consultants' views about the applicability of traditional theories and

---

[8] Where clinicians worked in major teaching hospitals in central London, for example, their expertise (in theory at least) would be available to all parties and some of these clinicians would accept instructions on both a local and a national basis. In practice, though, there was more overlap with regard to those experts instructed by the professional parties (i.e. the guardian, local authorities and the Official Solicitor) than with regard to experts instructed by professional parties and parents.

techniques in the assessment of Black and other ethnic minority children and parents.

Chapter 4 examines the impact of some of the major changes that Children Act proceedings have imposed on the work of the expert witness from the perspective of those on the receiving end – the experts themselves. It explores whether the quality of letters of instruction has improved, views about joint letters of instruction and the ethnical and practical issues these letters raise for child psychiatrists. This chapter also explores clinicians' views about the improvements made to their work as a consequence of the Children Act 1989.

In Chapter 5, in the light of concerns about what happens to child welfare knowledge once it is drawn into the legal arena, the study examined what might be termed 'the new clinical agenda', that is, the agenda for 'law' that is emerging from the work and views of those consultants who continue to work in this controversial field. Thus, questions are raised by experts about the ethical dilemmas that are emerging from this work, for example in making recommendations for treatment that other clinicians will usually have to take forward, and which locally based services may well struggle to provide, and with regard to the heavy weighting of resources in favour of a forensic exercise while clinical services before proceedings remained poor.

Equally, in the light of increased pressures on parties to adopt the use of joint letters of instruction to a single expert, child psychiatrists reflect on the implications of this trend both in terms of getting the best for highly vulnerable children, and with regard to indications for the real role of the child psychiatrist in public law litigation. Chapter 5 thus also explores views about competing expert evidence. It explores the advantages of the adversarial system, notions of what constitutes evidence, and views about meeting a known adversary in the legal arena. Finally, this chapter outlines the limitations and failures of Children Act proceedings from the perspective of child welfare specialists, looking at the lack of consistency of tribunals (i.e. judges and panels of magistrates) preparing cases for trial, lack of court powers to oversee treatment recommendations for children and the lack of feedback to and dialogue with these specialists.

Finally, Chapter 6 explores some of the implications for the family justice system of the changes to the role and responsibilities of the expert witness in child and family mental health. Some further changes in the training of specialist registrars and in social welfare policy initiatives since release for publication of the data reported in this book offer potential for improvements to some practices in this field. Thus, issues of collaboration and obligation are discussed in the light of new initiatives (e.g. Quality Protects programmes in local authority social services departments, and opportunities offered by the increased monies to the Child Mental Health Grant). Equally, a new edition of *Working Together* (Department of Health *et al*, 2000*b*) and a new *Framework for the Assessment of Children in Need and Their Families* (Department of Health *et al*, 2000*a*) offer some options for change. However, government plans for a further reorganisation of the National Health Service (NHS) (Department of Health, 2000) indicate a reduction in the time specialist registrars and consultants employed in the NHS may have for this type of work in the future. Thus the policy climate surrounding this work in Britain remains volatile and highly fragile.

# 1   The Children Act 1989: a new landscape for the work of expert witnesses

## The Act – a milestone in family proceedings

The Children Act 1989 was implemented on 14 October 1991. It aimed to revolutionise practice and proceedings concerning the welfare of children in England and Wales. The Act started from the principle that the primary responsibility for the upbringing of children rests with families, and that for most children their interests will be served best by enabling them to grow up in their own family. But changes brought about by the Act also reflected considerable concern and dissatisfaction with professional services for children following, for example, the Cleveland inquiry into child abuse and the deaths of children such as Jasmine Beckford, Kimberley Carlile and Doreen Aston while in their parents' care. Equally, the juvenile court was deemed inappropriate for care proceedings, as was also the dominance of a rescue over a preventive or respite approach to dealing with children considered to be at risk in their parents' care.

The Act therefore sought to achieve a better balance between reinforcing the autonomy of the family and enabling parents to exercise their parental responsibilities without state interference, and state support and protection of children where parents were failing or unable to meet their needs. Thus, it provided for support from local authorities for families where children were defined as 'in need',[1]

---

[1] Section 17 of the Children Act 1989 (local authority provision of services for children in need and their families), as outlined in *The Children Act Guidance and Regulations* (Department of Health, 1991*b*; see also Aldgate & Turnstill, 1996).

and also changed practice and procedures for the protection of children where there were concerns about child neglect or maltreatment. But the Children Act and its accompanying guidance (e.g. Department of Health, 1991*a,b*) did much more than simply change law and procedures for children deemed at risk: it also had implications for the work of all professionals and agencies involved in child protection work. It was not important simply because it was the first consolidating and comprehensive piece of legislation aimed at children and families for 50 years, but also because it was the outcome of a substantial amount of debate and public consultation about law, legal procedure and the philosophy and principles that should underscore changes in this field.[2]

The scope of the Children Act and its accompanying philosophy is extensive. It brought together both private and public law within one framework, it changed the structure and functioning of courts hearing family proceedings (see below),[3] and with regard to public law, importantly, it sought to achieve a better balance between the protection of children considered at risk and the need to ensure parents are able effectively to challenge state intervention. The aim was also to encourage greater partnership between statutory authorities and parents[4] and to promote the use of voluntary rather than compulsory arrangements between parents and local authorities wherever possible. Equally, the Act and guidance aimed to ensure that children and young people are consulted and are as fully informed as possible in actions and decisions about them. This is emphasised in the requirements for courts and professionals to consult with children and their parents and others and to take their wishes and views into consideration, and by giving children themselves the right to apply for court orders, and also by recognising in principle the rights of mature children to refuse consent to medical or psychiatric examinations. In addition, the Act and guidance recognised that issues of 'race', culture, language and religion are

---

[2] Several Law Commission papers on family law underscored the original Bill (e.g. Law Commission, 1986, 1987). The history of the public law aspects of the Act, beginning with the Short report (House of Commons, 1984) and the subsequent interdepartmental working party on child care law which reported in 1985 (Department of Health and Social Security, 1985), coincided with the production of working papers by the Law Commission and is reviewed by Ryan (1994, pp. 1–2).

[3] For example, although the Act failed to introduce a proper family court structure, it did introduce a 'concurrent jurisdiction' – see below.

[4] Although the word 'partnership' does not appear in the legislation and regulations, it did occur in government guidance on the Act and in the Department of Health's list of principles that should underpin practices (Department of Health, 1989, 1991*d*, 1995).

crucially important when courts and local authorities are making decisions about children.[5]

## The principles that guide the courts

The main principles that apply to all proceedings concerning the upbringing of children brought under the Act are:

(a) the child's welfare shall be the court's paramount consideration (section 1(1));
(b) a checklist of factors must be considered by courts when certain decisions are being made (section 1(3) – see below);
(c) delay in deciding questions concerning children is likely to prejudice their welfare (section 1(2));
(d) a court should not make an order under the Act with respect to a child unless it considers that making one would be better for the child than making no order at all (section 1(5)).

## A new court structure for family proceedings

### Concurrent jurisdiction

The relevant courts for cases under the Act are the magistrates' courts, which are called 'family proceedings courts' when hearing both private and public family law cases, the county courts (some of which are designated 'family hearing centres' for hearing private law applications, and a smaller number of which are designated 'care centres' for hearing public law applications), and the Family Division of the High Court.[6] Concurrent jurisdiction means that all these courts have the same powers regarding the range of orders available under the Act.

---

[5] Section 22(5)(c) and section 1(3) (the welfare checklist). Although there is no specific reference to race, culture, religion and language as such in the checklist, section 1(3)(d) does cover 'his age, sex, background and *any characteristics* [emphasis added] of his which the court considers relevant', thus arguably allowing for a consideration of these issues.

[6] In the family proceedings courts, all Children Act cases and other family proceedings are heard by magistrates from the court's family panel. These should consist of three justices with at least one man and one woman. With regard to the county court, there are three types of circuit judges nominated to deal with family proceedings. These are *designated* family judges (based at care centres and with full powers to deal with private and public law cases), *nominated* judges (also based at care centres and with full jurisdiction to hear private and public law cases) and *circuit* family judges (dealing with private law cases only).

Moreover, cases can be transferred to a higher court, a lower court or to another court at the same level (e.g. from one family proceedings court to another).[7]

## Court control

In both private and public law cases, the court is now required to establish a timetable for cases and to give directions for the preparation of cases to ensure that they are ready for a final hearing. Directions hearings were introduced, with two main purposes: to enable courts to exert control over the direction, substance and evidence in cases, and to deal with procedural issues to ensure cases are ready for the final hearing with a minimum of delay. Directions hearings are held in all tiers of the court structure. Practices may vary slightly depending on, for example, whether directions are complex or contested and whether they are being sought along with an interim application, but directions hearings generally take place before a district judge or circuit judge in the county court care centre and High Court, and before a justice's clerk in the family proceedings courts. However, if the issues for which direction of the court is sought are contested or complex, a directions hearing may be before a family panel of magistrates, stipendiary magistrate, or a district, county or High Court judge.

## Starting proceedings

The relevant court for beginning public law cases under the Children Act is the magistrates' family proceedings court.[8] But a case may be transferred to the relevant care centre[9] if the case is of exceptional gravity, importance or complexity, for example where there is or may be complicated or conflicting evidence or where there is a multiplicity of parties and cross-applications, or where a case raises an important point of law or public policy.[10] Also, a case may be transferred if there is a need to consolidate it with other proceedings, for example where proceedings concerning the child in question, or another child in

---

[7] Children (allocation of Proceedings) Order 1991 SI 1991/1677 (and later case law): the rules governing transfer are set out on p. 4.
[8] Unless they have been started as a result of a section 37 direction by a county court or High Court, or there are continuing public law proceedings concerning the same child going on in another court. In these circumstances proceedings should start in that court (article 3, Children (Allocation of Proceedings) Order 1991).
[9] Or the Principal Registry if the case emanates from the magistrates' family proceedings court serving the London boroughs.
[10] Article 18(3), Children (Allocation of Proceedings) Order 1991.

the same family, are underway in another court. In addition, it is also possible to transfer a case where this would 'significantly ... accelerate the hearing'.[11] Any party to proceedings can request that the case be transferred to a higher court, and a court can decide of its own volition to transfer a case.

## The guardian ad litem

In all specified proceedings (i.e. all public law applications, including those to place children in secure accommodation and applications for emergency protection orders) the court must appoint a guardian ad litem for the child 'unless it is not necessary to do so in order to safeguard his interests' (section 41(1)). This appointment should take place as soon as possible following a court application. The background and the development of the role and duties of the guardian ad litem following the Children Act 1989 are outlined and discussed by Brophy & Bates (1999, p. 7).[12] In brief, guardians are under a duty to safeguard the interests of the child and they appoint and instruct a solicitor to act on behalf of the child.[13] They have to act in accordance with the welfare principle – the child's welfare is paramount – and with the principle that delay is prejudicial to children. Guardians also have to consider all the factors in the welfare checklist (see below) when carrying out their duties. In addition, as officers of the court, guardians are under a duty to advise the court on matters such as timetabling, the appropriate court for hearing a case, the use of expert evidence, the wishes and feelings of children and a child's level of understanding, for example in consenting to medical examinations. Equally, guardians advise the court of the options available to it and the suitability of each option.

Guardians investigate the background to the case and read the local authority files to scrutinise the local authority's conduct of the case. They also have the right to copy any documents relevant to the child and are under a duty to attend all directions hearings unless excused by the court.[14] They can be asked to produce interim reports during proceedings and they must produce a final report, which must be served on other parties to proceedings.[15]

---

[11] Article 7(1), Children (Allocation of Proceedings) Order 1991.
[12] And national standards for the work of the guardian were introduced by the Department of Health (1996).
[13] Unless a child wishes to instruct a solicitor him- or herself and is considered of sufficient understanding to do this.
[14] Rule 11(6), section 42, and rule 11(4).
[15] Rule 11 (7).

Thus, the guardian's role is extensive, and the work of the guardian was, and is, seen as crucial to the success of the Children Act. Their duties and responsibilities involve both reflecting back and looking forward. The former (investigative) task entails examining how child protection and family support work have been organised by a local authority with a particular family. This includes interviewing such persons as the guardian thinks appropriate[16] (or as directed by the court). It also entails an examination of local authority records and an assessment, for example, of the extent to which a local authority has attempted to work in consultation and partnership with a family on a voluntary basis, thus alleviating the need for compulsory intervention. It will also entail examining the degree to which a child and parents have cooperated with statutory agencies. Moreover, since court rules make special provision regarding an examination or an assessment of a child – no child may be seen by an expert for the purposes of preparing a report for the proceedings without permission of the court[17] – the guardian has to consider at an early stage in proceedings whether there is any need for expert assessments or examinations. The guardian is thus expected to play a full and active role, not only as the representative and spokesperson for the child, but also as an adviser to the court on both procedural and evidential issues.

## Local authority support for children and families

Part III and schedule 2 of the Children Act 1989 deal with local authority support for children and their families and it outlines a range of duties and powers for local authorities with regard to the provision of services for children 'in need'. So, for example, it details the law regarding the provision of accommodation for children by local authorities and introduces the new concept of children being 'looked after' by the local authority. This term now applies to children who come into local authority care either voluntarily (i.e. as a result of choice by parents or children) or as a result of statutory intervention resulting in a care order under section 31 of the Act (see below).

The background to the term 'family support', which was used in the government's *Review of Child Care Law* (Department of Health and Social

---

[16] Guardians must decide how detailed their enquiries should be, but the list includes not simply parents and other adults who are important to the child – it also extends to any siblings, members of the child's extended family and other professionals such as health visitors, general practitioners, school teachers, and so on.

[17] FPC (CA 1989) R 1991 r 18(1); FPR 1991 r 14 18(1).

Security, 1985), and the development of the duties of the local authority to provide services to prevent the need for children to come into care are reviewed by Ryan (1994, pp. 23–57), as are the child protection procedures undertaken by local authorities before the instigation of care proceedings (pp. 59–72). That background provides the framework for understanding the role of the guardian ad litem not only in assessing the extent and quality of the pre-court work undertaken by local authorities, but also in reviewing the need for any additional specialist assessments beyond those of social workers, for example by child psychiatrists.

Under the Act, local authorities have a general duty:

> "(a) to safeguard and promote the welfare of children within their
>     area who are in need, and
> (b) so far as is consistent with that duty, to promote the upbringing
>     of such children by their families,
> by providing a range and level of services appropriate to those
> children's needs." (Section 17(1)).

The general duty embodies two important principles underlying the Act: first, the desire to have legislation that positively promotes family support work; and second, the belief that the welfare of the majority of children will be safeguarded best by enabling them to grow up within their own family. Because local authorities have a duty to reduce the need to initiate care or supervision proceedings, when they are considering making an application for a care or supervision order (see below), whether in the context of existing court proceedings or as part of a child protection investigation, they must consider what other options might be available (para. 7, schedule 2 of the Act). In other words, a care or supervision order should be sought only where there appears to be no better way of safeguarding and promoting the welfare of the child; thus, voluntary arrangements through the provision of services to the child and family should always be fully explored (Department of Health, 1991a, para. 3.2).

## Proceedings for care and supervision applications

Part IV of the Children Act 1989 deals with disputes between parents and the state regarding the care and upbringing of children. Many of the changes introduced by the Act were a response to sustained criticism about the complexities, anomalies and injustices of previous legislation. For example, as outlined by Ryan (1994, p. 97): children could come into proceedings via a variety of routes, with varying criteria for entry; the legal position of children differed depending on which route had brought them into care; local authorities could assume parental rights by an administrative procedure; children, parents and other relatives were unable to challenge local authority decisions about contact with children in care – save in limited circumstances; and there was unequal access to the wardship jurisdiction of the High Court.

Most of these anomalies and injustices were tackled by the Children Act in an attempt to achieve a better balance between the needs of children for protection and the rights of parents to participate fully in proceedings – even though some new problems have emerged (see Brophy & Bates, 1998). Thus, under section 31(1), only the local authority or an 'authorised' person (e.g. the National Society for the Prevention of Cruelty to Children (NSPCC) or any of its officers – section (9)(a)) can make an application for a care or supervision order and the local authority can no longer use the inherent jurisdiction of the High Court for such purposes. Parents are able to challenge local authority decisions, children are separately represented, the guardian ad litem reviews the work undertaken by the local authority with a child and parents and makes recommendations in respect of the paramount welfare of the child, and where members of the extended family have a distinct interest in the proceedings they can apply to the court to become parties in proceedings.

Under section 31(2), the Children Act sets out a single set of conditions that must be established before the court can consider whether to make an order under the Act. These conditions, called the threshold criteria, are:

" (a)  That the child concerned is suffering, or likely to suffer, significant harm, and
  (b)  That the harm or likelihood of harm, is attributable to –
     (i)   That care given to the child, or likely to be given to him were the order not made, not being what it would be reasonable to expect a parent to give him; or
     (ii)  That the child's being beyond parental control."

## The 'significant harm' criteria

The definition of 'harm' in the Act, defined by section 31(9), centres on ill treatment or the impairment of health or development. 'Ill treatment' is defined as including sexual and physical abuse and forms of ill treatment that are not physical (e.g. mental). Impairment of health or development can also provide the basis of 'harm'. 'Health' is defined as physical or mental health, while 'development' is defined as physical, intellectual, emotional or behavioural development. White (1998) usefully defined the thinking and assessment exercise

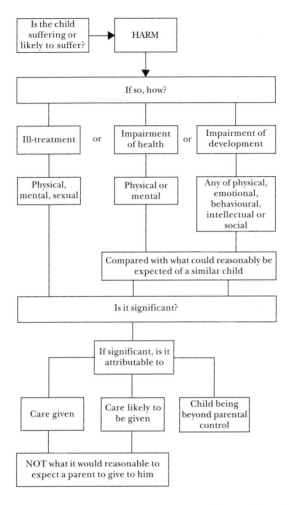

*Fig. 1. The criteria for significant harm. Source: White (1998, p. 19); with permission.*

indicated by the criteria for significant harm in terms of a series of 'steps'. These are shown in a flow diagram in Fig. 1.

While there was no definition of 'significant' when the Bill was debated, the Lord Chancellor said, "It speaks of significant harm – namely that which, being more than minimal, indicates that compulsory care or supervision may be justified".[18] In early guidance, the Department of Health (1991*a*, para. 3.21) argued that "minor

---

[18] Hansard, House of Lords, 19 January 1989, col. 343.

shortcomings in health care or minor deficits in physical, psychological or social development should not require compulsory intervention unless cumulatively they are having, or are likely to have, serious and lasting effects upon the child".

Where the facts relate to health or development, it is also necessary to compare the health or development with what could reasonably be expected of a similar child (section 31(10)). This test has raised several questions about interpretation of 'a similar child'; for example, Ryan (1994) and White (1991) questioned whether a different test might apply depending on demographic, socio-economic and ethnic status.[19]

The threshold conditions require evidence on two issues before they can be established. The first is establishing the existence, or likely existence, of significant harm at the date of the commencement of the protective proceedings, and the second is establishing that the harm is attributable to a lack of reasonable parental care. The court must then go on to consider the welfare principle, and to determine whether or not the order would be better for the child than no order at all (section 1(5)). In considering what order to make, the court is instructed to have regard in particular to a welfare checklist set out in section 1(3)):

(a) the ascertainable wishes and feelings of the child concerned (considered in the light of his age and understanding);
(b) his physical, emotional and educational needs;
(c) the likely effect on him of any change in his circumstances;
(d) his age, sex, background and any characteristics of his which the court considers relevant;
(e) any harm which he has suffered or is at risk of suffering;
(f) how capable each of his parents, and any other person in relation to whom the court considered the question to be relevant, is of meeting his needs;
(g) the powers available to the court under this Act in the proceedings in question.

## A new landscape for experts

The above changes to law and legal procedure and the philosophies on which these changes were based presented a new and very different

---

[19] The Department of Health (1991*a*, para. 3.20) argued that the meaning of 'similar' in this context would be a matter of judicial interpretation but that it might take account of the environmental, social and cultural characteristics of the child.

landscape for the work of expert witnesses in child proceedings. But few people could have envisaged the increased reliance of courts and local authorities on the expertise of health professionals (cf. Adcock, 1991, p. 12). Some clinicians (e.g. Bentovim, 1991 *a,b*; Jones *et al*, 1991; Lau, 1991; Lynch, 1991)[20] did begin to address the concept of significant harm, and what constituted 'abuse', 'normal' development and 'impairment'. In the context of discussing resources in general, Morrison (1991, p. 88) was somewhat prophetic in reviewing research on the treatment of 'abusing parents' and arguing that knowledge and research in this field would be essential for the future work of courts. He argued that "we will need to assess more quickly who is treatable". But no writers, policy makers or clinicians addressed the question of demand relative to possible supply of clinical services for litigation purposes either before or shortly after implementation of the Act.

As the Children Act bedded in, two things were clear. First, the benchmark, set by the Children Act Advisory Committee (1991/2, p. 2) in its first *Annual Report*, of some 12 weeks for completing proceedings was quickly demonstrated to be totally unrealistic – even those cases that started and ended in the family proceedings courts and that did not involve any expert evidence did not meet this deadline (Bates & Brophy, 1996, table 31). Second, the demand for clinical assessments – especially from child psychiatrists – presented substantial problems not only of supply (Children Act Advisory Committee, 1993/4, pp. 14–15) but also, in some instances, of quality (Brophy & Bates, 1998).

## *The use of experts following the Children Act 1989*

Two studies on the use of expert evidence in care and related proceedings provided the foundations for the study presented in this book (Bates & Brophy, 1996; Brophy *et al*, 1999*b*). These studies provided a range of findings about the use of experts generally (i.e. across all disciplines and by all parties) and about the use of local CAMHS in particular. For example, Brophy *et al* included a national random survey of cases involving expert evidence. The sample consisted of 557 cases concerning just under 1000 children. There were six major findings. First, reports from child psychiatrists formed the dominant type of expert evidence commissioned – these reports appeared in some 41% of all cases.[21] Second, this was the major source

---

[20] In the early 1990s Lau (1991) was one of the few child psychiatrists to consider the concept of significant harm with specific regard to Black and other ethnic minority groups in Britain (cf. Maitra, 1995, 1996).

of evidence commissioned by the professional parties (i.e. the local authority and the guardian ad litem). Third, parents were much less likely to file reports from child psychiatrists and more likely to file reports from adult psychiatrists.[22] Fourth, it was very unusual for 'medical' evidence, that is, evidence from paediatricians, paediatric radiologists and so on, to be the only evidence in cases (under 11% of cases); rather, this evidence was generally followed by evidence commissioned from child psychiatrists.[23] Fifth, most child psychiatrists undertaking assessments for litigation purposes were working alone: 41% of cases contained reports from a single clinician, while only 15% contained a multi-disciplinary report. Finally – and contrary to much received wisdom at the time – most cases in the survey did not contain expert evidence filed by all three major parties in the proceedings: only 18% of cases fell into this category (Brophy *et al*, 1999*b*, figure 4.1).

The national survey also explored guardians' views on and use of 'locally' based CAMHS, the problems they were encountering, the improvements they wished to see in services and the criteria they applied in selecting a child psychiatrist. Relatively few guardians were satisfied with locally based CAMHS in so far as these services were able/willing to provide assessments and reports for courts – no guardian was unreservedly satisfied, while only 19% said they were mostly satisfied with services.[24] Of those who expressed dissatisfaction:

(a) 72% were critical of local services because they lacked resources or a commitment to undertake further therapeutic work with children if that was deemed necessary;

---

[21] This compares with paediatric reports filed in 35% of all cases; psychiatric reports on parent(s) filed in 32%; and psychological reports on parents and children filed in 12% (Brophy *et al*, 1999*b*, table 4.9).

[22] Where parents were the only party to file any expert evidence in cases, psychiatric reports based on *adults only* appeared in over half (54%). Where parents were one of a number of parties to file any evidence, adult psychiatric reports appeared in 33% of cases. In contrast, parents filed *child and family* psychiatric reports in 12% and 15% of cases respectively (Brophy *et al*, 1999*b*, table 4.9).

[23] This is not of course to suggest that psychiatrists are not medically trained but rather to differentiate the disciplines that may be commissioned in proceedings. These disciplines and specialist fields are outlined in detail by Brophy *et al* (1999*b*, table 4.9).

[24] The response rate for the national survey of guardians was 71%; 31% of respondents were not satisfied with the service provided by the local CAMHS, and 50% said it was variable and depended on the area (Brophy *et al*, 1999*b*, p. 12).

(b) 63% were also critical of local services because they lacked staff with sufficient training and experience to undertake instructions in public law proceedings;

(c) 59% were critical of local services because of delays in getting reports.

In other words, the major sources of complaint were generated by the lack of a comprehensive service for children who are abused, neglected or otherwise maltreated by parents.

Among the improvements that guardians wished to see from the CAMHS were more locally based services able to work in this field and offer ongoing help to children, more resources and more staff trained and experienced in public law work, and an increase in the availability of multi-disciplinary teams able to offer a range of skills and expertise. Interestingly, while guardians were critical of many local CAMHS, they tended to be satisfied with the experts they themselves instructed: 88% were satisfied with the experts they used. The reason for most of the discrepancy (between assessments of local CAMHS and the clinicians instructed by guardians) was that, in certain sectors of the country at least, guardians tended not to use local services but rather tried to instruct a relatively small cadre of experts who were willing to work on a national basis.[25]

Moreover, the findings also demonstrated that, in selecting an expert, guardians have two priorities. First, they require a clinician with a particular understanding of and sympathy with the needs of children *and* families involved in public law proceedings – not all clinicians were seen as 'user-friendly' in this regard. Second, clinicians must have previous experience as an expert witness and this included being skilled in the witness box and able to withstand cross-examination. In other words, the 'tried and trusted' expert dominated appointments. But guardians were also aware of the range of difficulties for child psychiatrists. They were aware of the anxieties that court work can provoke in untrained and inexperienced clinicians and of the reluctance of some therefore to get involved in cases. As Table 10 (p. 102) shows, some clinicians have posed a lack of time and general work overload as reasons for not undertaking instructions, some saw a conflict of interests between their clinical work and court work, but others expressed an unwillingness to be 'grilled' in court or to expose their work to criticism (Brophy *et al*, 1999*b*, p. 16).

---

[25] That is, clinicians who did not restrict instructions to a geographical area but who were willing to accept instruction on a national basis.

This, then, was the new and dynamic landscape for expert witnesses instructed in public law under the Children Act in the 1990s. 'Law' (case law, reports and practice directions from the Children Act Advisory Committee) increasingly attempted to control and regulate the agenda for the use of experts by setting out the duties and responsibilities for advocates instructing experts, for courts when giving parties leave (i.e. permission) to instruct experts and for experts themselves when undertaking assessments within legal proceedings.[26] Advocates were instructed to consider whether a joint appointment of one expert might be achievable, whether expert evidence in any given category could be adduced by one party, and whether and why experts in the same discipline needed to be instructed by more than one party. When seeking leave to appoint an expert, advocates were also instructed to provide the court with full information on the category of expert required, the focus of the assessment, the need for the evidence and the relevance of expert evidence to the issues under discussion.

In theory at least, the days of 'here are the papers, tell us what you think' were over. When writing the letter of instruction, advocates were told to set out the context in which the opinion was requested and to define specific questions to be addressed by the expert. The loss of litigation privilege in Children Act cases means that whatever the content of the resulting report, this now has to be disclosed to other parties and to the court. Advocates were also told to disclose the letter of instruction to other parties and to include it in the bundle of documents submitted to the court. In granting leave for expert evidence, courts were instructed there should be no 'blanket' leave for paper opinions, that they should routinely enquire into the category of expert required, the relevance of the evidence requested, whether a joint instruction was possible and whether one party only (particularly the guardian ad litem) could commission the expert, and, when granting leave for a second opinion, that they should enquire why there was a need for more than one expert of the same discipline. In addition, courts were instructed to give directions as to the timescale in which the evidence should be produced,[27] the disclosure of resultant

---

[26] For example, early case law – particularly *Re R (A Minor) (Expert's Evidence)* [1991] 1 FLR 291; *Re J (Child Abuse: Expert Evidence)* [1991] FCR 193; *Re AB (Child Abuse: Expert Witnesses)* [1994] 1 FLR 181; *Re G (Minors) (Expert Witnesses)* [1994] 2 FLR 291) – practice directions (The President's Practice Direction on Case Management [1995] 1 FLR 456), and the Children Act Advisory Committee (1991/2, 1992/3, 1993/4, 1994/5, 1995/6, 1996/7, 1997), as well as Booth (1996) all sought to modify and improve practices in this field.

[27] Or if, at the time of granting leave, that was impractical, to set a date for those directions to be given.

reports to other parties and, if there was a conflict of expert opinion, the discussions that should take place between experts and the filing of a statement identifying areas of agreement and disagreement.

Experts in turn were instructed not to be partisan, to provide a straightforward and not misleading opinion and not to mislead by omission; reports should be properly researched (indicating areas of insufficient data) and should clearly state if the report is provisional. Also, experts were instructed to maintain accuracy in the dating of reports and to stick to the brief given by the court.

This was the new terrain that was being carved, in effect a new interface between 'law' and the work of child welfare specialists. New research (e.g. Bates & Brophy, 1996; Brophy *et al*, 1999*b*; Hunt & Macleod, 1998) and case law following the Children Act 1989 demonstrated the interdisciplinary nature of proceedings and the central role of child psychiatrists in that development. But the perspective of experts themselves was missing. Contemporary debate raised questions about their work and the value of their contributions, but few contributors questioned what it might be like to be 'on the receiving end' of a very much more prescriptive but rapidly changing legal agenda. Equally, the lack of policy initiatives on the part of central government to deal with the supply if not the training aspects of CAMHS provision during the 1990s was striking. Chapters 2–5 therefore aim to demonstrate how experts themselves responded to the issues and challenges posed by allegations of child abuse/neglect within the framework posed by Children Act proceedings.

# 2 NHS structures and contracts: the context in which child psychiatrists meet the needs set by care proceedings

## Introduction

Although legal discourses continued to set out a new agenda for the work of child welfare specialists during the 1990s, little attention was given to the institutional and contractual framework within which consultants responded to that challenge. Moreover, there has been little systematic examination of how those structures might influence the availability and willingness of individual specialists to undertake assessments and provide reports within child protection litigation.

Below, therefore, the public law work of a sample of consultants is explored in the light of the NHS reforms to the provision of community health services introduced by the NHS and Community Care Act 1990. The question of waiting lists for medico-legal work is addressed along with some of the dilemmas that are raised for consultants who are asked to undertake forensic work with families for whom they already have a clinical responsibility. Finally, the question of how often consultants might meet with children and parents when undertaking assessments is explored, and there is a review of the length of experience respondents had at consultant level within their profession and as expert witnesses.

# From welfare state to welfare markets?
# Medico-legal work during the NHS reforms at the
# beginning of the 1990s

The funding and delivery of the public law sections of medico-legal work are extremely complex. The contractual obligations of individual child psychiatrists in this respect appear to have been slightly clearer before the introduction of the market model and contracting with the NHS and Community Care Act 1990.[1] Before these reforms, broadly speaking, consultants had a contract with a health authority for work related to the diagnosis, treatment or prevention of illness of NHS patients. This was deemed to be 'category 1' work in terms of service provision; it was free at the point of delivery, but it usually excluded medico-legal work.[2] Prior to the NHS and Community Care Act 1990, medico-legal work could be undertaken by consultants on maximum part-time contracts in the context of what was termed 'category 2' work and for which a fee might be charged (and this option persists). However, it appears that doctors with full-time NHS contracts

---

[1] The framework for state intervention was extensively recast by legislative and contractual changes. The NHS and Community Care Act 1990 separated the commissioning of services from their provision, particularly in the health services, changing the emphasis from the provision of services to the meeting of needs (Audit Commission, 1994, p. 6, para. 8).

[2] This being one of a range of services for which doctors can charge a fee. The Private Practice and Professional Fees Committee of the British Medical Association (BMA) negotiates and suggests a range of fees to cover many of these services. Doctors must ensure that in levying a charge they do not have an obligation to provide the service without a charge under their contract or terms of service. The contractual duties of hospital doctors in the NHS are contained in individual contracts of which the *Terms and Conditions of Service for Hospital Medical Staff* may form part. In broad terms, the level of fee charged for a service depends on who pays and how it is determined. The BMA groups fees into four categories. Those fees under what is termed category D in the BMA schedule (i.e. where fees are not prescribed by statute or negotiated nationally with, for example, government departments or local authorities under categories A–C) should be "agreed between the doctor and party concerned". The BMA provides some guidance for doctors in determining their own professional fees for non-NHS services but they are not "recommended fees". As the BMA acknowledges with regard to hospital doctors, the dividing line between work they can or cannot charge for is blurred (British Medical Association, 1996, para. 4.4.2). As outlined above, for the most part, where consultant psychiatrists undertake public law work (and depending on their own contracts and the existence of any agreements under BMA category B) this work, or part of it, is likely to be undertaken as category 2 work under the doctor's individual contract of service – for which they may charge a fee. The government subsequently proposed changes to the NHS in July 2000, which may amend aspects of this contract (Department of Health, 2000) – see Chapter 6.

were nevertheless also free to undertake a certain amount of private work and thus could also undertake some medico-legal work.

Bailey (1995) pointed out conflicts of interest between consultants' work within the NHS and that outside it. He argues that consultants with a full-time NHS contract are nevertheless free to undertake private practice at any time, and many have contracts that allow them to do as much private work as they wish, as long as they "devote substantially the whole of their professional time to the NHS" (subject presumably to the "10%" rule – see below). There appears to be no independent data to allow assessment of whether the extent of consultants' private practice has an effect on their ability to meet their contractual NHS commitments, although Bailey reports that it is possible to examine the relation between private practice and the *amount* of work carried out for the NHS. He states (1995, p. 790) that "although most consultants do not do private work at the expense of the NHS, the 25 per cent of full-time consultants doing the most private work tend to do significantly less NHS work than their colleagues". Although Bailey's work on the changing role of hospital doctors did not include child psychiatrists, there are no reasons to suppose that their contracts differ from those of consultants in public health medicine and community health generally and, thus, the rule that doctors with full-time contracts may earn up to 10% of their gross full-time salary income from private practice would apply (British Medical Association, 1996, p. 11, para. 5.5).[3]

In essence, it appears that, whether working part time or full time, doctors were absolutely free to choose whether or not they undertook medico-legal work and whether, within that broad field, they undertook any public law work. In practice, with regard to public law work for local authorities, the dividing line between what could and what could not be chargeable at the point of delivery was somewhat blurred. For example, in certain instances where letters of instruction came from a local authority, it appears that the clinical assessment was undertaken as part of the NHS contract, but writing up the report and, if necessary, appearing in court to give evidence, would be costed separately as category 2 work. The organisation of the public law commitments of some consultants in this study conformed to this model.

There was a further blurring of contractual boundaries following the 1990 NHS reforms. It appeared that some NHS trusts, in joint commissioning arrangements with local authorities, set up contracts

---

[3] But see note 2 above and Chapter 6 regarding proposed changes to doctors' contracts within the NHS.

with consultants which specified that a consultant would carry out a number of pieces of medico-legal work for a local authority in one year, that is, under category 1 work and, thus, free at the point of delivery.

Data from these interviews indicated that, at the time of the study, the picture at the interface between purchasers of expert evidence (i.e. local authorities, but also guardians and parents) and providers of that service (i.e. consultants in medicine and psychiatry) was, to say the least, diverse. The nature of contractual obligations between local authorities and local NHS trusts, and between NHS trusts and individual consultants employed with those services, was extremely complex and remained, for many, in a state of transition. New arrangements announced by a Labour government in 1997 (aimed at breaking down barriers between health and social services departments: see Chapter 6), coupled with the recommendations of the Audit Commission (1999) for improved effectiveness and efficiency of CAMHS, indicate that states of transition in this field are likely to persist for some considerable time. The practices outlined below, therefore, in terms of employment base/contractual obligations of the consultants, may not be a completely comprehensive picture of the way in which child psychiatrists undertake assessments and reports for courts in public law proceedings either at the time of the study or as a consequence of subsequent changes.[4] However, the interviews highlighted some of the most important practices that underscore how this work is provided and thus indicate the issues that require further discussion in order to develop CAMHS to meet the needs of courts addressing neglected and maltreated children and their parents in the twenty-first century.

## Custom and practice or contractual obligation? The work of the child psychiatrist in child protection litigation

The difficulties outlined above of trying to untangle both the history of the extra-contractual aspects of the work of child psychiatrists and the situation pertaining at the time the interviews were undertaken were well summarised by one national consultant interviewed:

---

[4] Nor would they necessarily apply to all experts in proceedings. For example, in looking at the supply situation in relation to clinical or educational psychologists, one would need to explore the ways in which the institutional base and personal contracts influence the ability or willingness of these professionals to accept public law referrals both within and outside the NHS.

TABLE 1
*Institutional/employment base of the 17 consultants in the study*

| Location | 'National' experts (n = 6) | 'Local' experts (n = 11) |
|---|---|---|
| Clinical post in an NHS trust | 2 | 10 |
| Academic post in a medical school or teaching hospital | 2 | 1 |
| Retired or semi-retired | 2 | 0 |

> "If anybody tells you that contracts within the NHS are clearly defined and well organised, don't believe them! What is in a contract or not in a contract is as vague as vague can be. By custom and practice we have done a certain number of court reports on an NHS basis for the local authority ... but it's true to say that in [this area] it's only Dr 'Smith' and I who are still doing court reports as NHS cases. Everybody else has got so frustrated with the system that they've just said no, we won't do it any more." (N12)

Despite the complexity described by consultants regarding how and when they undertook court work, some broad patterns emerged from the sample. It is important to begin by looking at the institutional/ employment base and how working agendas were organised, because to a large extent this determined the way in which referrals for assessments and reports within public law proceedings were accommodated. Table 1 gives a breakdown of the institutional settings of the sample.

The great majority of 'local' experts in this sample held a clinical post in an NHS trust, but some (just under half) also had research and teaching responsibilities. The institutional bases of the 'national' experts indicated there may be considerably more variation in the employment status of this group of consultants. In this sample, they were evenly divided among the three possible employment/institutional locations identified in Table 1. Thus, a few of the national experts were either retired or semi-retired from mainstream NHS clinical work and were undertaking court work privately.[5] The main task of the national experts with academic posts was teaching at under- and postgraduate level, along with some research and some clinical work for a trust.

---

[5] It should also be noted that, in certain contexts, referrals for assessments during litigation could be undertaken by a consultant as a means of generating extra income for a trust.

TABLE 2
*Contracts and patterns of accommodation of public law work*

| Contract | Pattern of accommodation |
| --- | --- |
| Private work | Some consultants (those who were retired/ semi-retired from NHS) undertook referrals on a private basis |
| Chargeable as category 2 work | Some consultants who remained in NHS employment continued to undertake the majority of their court work under category 2 of their terms and conditions of employment |
| Mainstream NHS category 1 work | Some consultants were undertaking assessments for court proceedings as part of their NHS contract of employment and did not do any extra-contractual work in this field (i.e. no private work, no category 2 work) |
| Combination of category 1 and category 2 work | Some consultants did court work only where proceedings arose in ongoing NHS treatment of children and families; where this happened part of the subsequent task could be undertaken (and charged for) as category 2 work |

It may be the case, therefore, that some consultants on the 'national network'[6] play a larger role in ongoing research and teaching than do consultants working in clinical posts in NHS trusts. But it is probably also the case that a number of national experts will have retired completely from clinical practice within the NHS. These consultants may perhaps undertake some limited teaching, but overall may be less likely to undertake any further significant research. However, as one such consultant in this study argued, they certainly have considerably more time to read published research than when they headed a busy and increasingly overstretched clinical deparment.

Looking at the institutional location of clinicians providing assessments and reports for public law proceedings, a number of issues are apparent. First, although there was considerable variety in the way in which consultants undertook assessments and reports for courts in care proceedings, discussions about how court work fits in with other responsibilities indicated some distinct patterns of accommodation (Table 2).

Very few consultants in this sample were contracted to provide local authorities with assessments and reports for courts as part of their

---

[6] It is important in this debate constantly to keep in mind the very small number of consultants undertaking this type of work – see note 5 in Chapter 1.

mainstream NHS contracted work and some consultants indicated that there was resistance to making court work part of their mainstream responsibilities within the NHS.

For those consultants undertaking this type of work from an institutional base, most of it was carried out as 'category 2' work. Consultants offered varying definitions and understandings of that category:

> "It's work that you are not contracted to do. You don't have to do it ... and it mustn't interfere with your NHS commitments." (L19)

> "There is a clear distinction that the contract permits you to use your expertise, not to treat patients, but to offer advice to insurance companies, solicitors, and courts in an independent manner – but that is not regarded as private practice." (L8)

In those apparently limited areas where the NHS reforms of 1990 resulted in some trusts jointly commissioning CAMHS with local authorities such that consultants had a contract that specified a certain number of pieces of court work for the local authority, the study identified that this change had not been without its problems. For example, in services that continued to be characterised by a chronic lack of resources there were problems about how to prioritise this new category of (medico-legal) work. For the most part, assessments and reports for courts in care proceedings had a low clinical priority compared with other types of referrals, for example deliberate self-harm, anorexic and acutely disturbed children. Thus, in the final analysis, whatever the contracted obligation, a new referral from a local authority in the context of legal proceedings would not be accepted by a consultant if there were other children whom the consultant considered should have a higher clinical priority, or, indeed, if the instructions received from a local authority were of poor quality:

> "People keep going back to a commitment under section 27[7] but the problem is that an agreement between a health authority and a local authority appears to forget the fact that at the sharp end there's a chap who's actually got to do the job. It's not the local authority who does the job or the health authority, it's me, as the consultant psychiatrist, and I don't care what agreement a health authority has come to with the local authority, if a local authority asks me to do a job which I consider to be impossible, unjust, badly thought out, badly constructed I will say no. So that whole business

---

[7] Section 27 of the Children Act 1989, under which the then area health authority was one of a number of agencies asked to assist the local authority in providing services to children in need.

needs to be looked at very carefully. It's a fundamental flaw in the thinking that's gone into the current purchaser–provider split in the NHS, that a purchaser can say 'Yes, we'll purchase this service' – without determining whether the provider can actually provide it." (N12)

Two issues were clear from these interviews. First, individual choice based on consultants' clinical autonomy determined whether this type of work was undertaken. Second, most consultants reported they were undertaking this work outside their NHS practice, most of it, they argued, being undertaken in the evenings and at weekends.[8] In the movement towards an internal market in the NHS, it appeared that assessments and reports for care proceedings were not, on the whole, viewed as part of the essential core services that many CAMHS were contracted to supply for local authorities.

The exclusion of medico-legal work in general from mainstream NHS work is not a new practice. However, following the Children Act 1989, it is necessary to place these findings in a new context. Historically CAMHS have been neglected and under-resourced – the Cinderella of the NHS (Trowell, 1991, p. 14; Association of Directors of Social Services & Royal College of Psychiatrists, 1995/6). Thus, services have always been, to say the least, somewhat 'patchy' (House of Commons Health Committee, 1997, para. 14). More recently a survey of CAMHS undertaken by the Audit Commission (1999) found that one in five children suffers from mental health problems, but specialist services within mainstream NHS provision suffer substantial problems (Box 1).

---

Box 1
*Are CAMHS meeting the health needs of children and families?*
*Some results of an Audit Commission survey*

- Inequalities in the distribution of services around the country.
- Substantial variations in expenditure per child (a ratio of 7:1), with little relation to local needs.
- Substantial variation in the mix of staff deployed in services.
- Poor local links with other services, with only 2% of specialist staff time allocated to providing consultation services.
- Very few referrals (14%) from social services departments.
- Very few trusts (about 10%) could offer a non-urgent appointment within 6 months.
- Only half of health authorities had agreements for emergency 24-hour cover.
- Over one-third of trusts felt they could not respond effectively to young people presenting in a crisis.

Source: Audit Commission (1999).

---

[8] Court appearances, however, would not be possible outside of normal working hours.

Nevertheless, over the past decade there has been a substantial rise in referrals for assessments within the context of public law proceedings (Brophy *et al*, 1999*b*, pp. 5–7). This rise has been coupled with a redefinition of the tasks and an extension of duties expected of clinicians acting as expert witnesses. However, these changes occurred at a time when reductions in budget and staffing meant that many CAMHS were facing a crisis in their ability to provide even the traditional, contracted core services to the community.[9] A marked feature of this reduction in resources that is of particular importance for public law litigation has been the loss of multi-disciplinary teams in some areas (Trowell, 1991; Sepping, 1992; Tufnell & Seymour, 1993).

In other words, the demands of 'law' for services from child health specialists increased in both volume and complexity at a time when many clinical services were in fact being reduced as result of chronic under-funding relative to community need. However, it should also be remembered that the provision and funding of much of this work (if not the expertise) appeared to fall outside of core NHS services.

## Waiting lists for medico-legal work

Where consultants were working from an institutional base and undertaking instructions in public law proceedings as category 2 work, because of the way in which they organised and prioritised their work (i.e. clinical cases taking priority), there was unlikely to be a specific waiting list for children and families requiring assessments and reports for public law proceedings. At the point of enquiry by an advocate representing a party, if consultants had time and could meet the deadline set for filing the report, they would on the whole accept the instructions;[10] otherwise, they would simply turn the request down and the advocate would have to search elsewhere.

---

[9] See also Association of Directors of Social Services & Royal College of Psychiatrists (1995/6, pp. 4–6), House of Commons Health Committee (1997, para. 14), NHS Executive, North West Regional Office (1997, pp. 12–16), NHS Health Advisory Service (1995, pp. 11–13). Attempts to improve the national coverage of CAHMS underscored a grant of £84 million over three years to children's mental health in 1999; however, none of this new money was specifically earmarked for work in child protection litigation – see Chapter 6.

[10] Some consultants included criteria such as whether a case was of interest to their particular field of clinical practice or research, the need to stagger work that involved child sexual abuse, because of its emotional impact, and the need to ensure sufficient distance between cases so as not to confuse issues and feelings arising from different cases. Many consultants were also reluctant to undertake instructions on behalf of parents.

# Working practices: working alone or in a multi-disciplinary team

All consultants undertaking assessments and reports for public law proceedings either privately or as category 2 work (the majority of consultants in this study) were, in effect, working alone. This finding is in line with that obtained from the national survey discussed in Chapter 1 (41% of cases contained reports from a single child psychiatrist compared with 15% of cases containing a multi-disciplinary report – Brophy *et al*, 1999*b*). However, the practices of those consultants undertaking this work as part of their contract of employment indicated a mixture of both team work and individual work.

Those few consultants who *only* undertook this type of work within the context of contracted work within a trust (i.e. those doing no court work under category 2 of their contract) tended to work in a multi-disciplinary team of specialists. This was largely because they were responsible for managing a team of people either available to work on cases or already working on cases in which the children subsequently became the subject of legal proceedings. However, as the Audit Commission (1999) also later found, multi-disciplinary assessments for court proceedings were less possible than five years previously. Consultants stated that this was due to reductions in staffing levels in units and the loss of other team members. Thus, for example, one consultant stated that he now undertook assessments of children and parents for legal proceedings alone – he said they were quicker, but not as good as when undertaken by a multi-disciplinary team.[11] Another consultant, discussing negotiations about future 'purchaser' needs, said the local authority involved had yet to decide whether it wished to remain with a single psychiatrist, or whether it wished to purchase a multi-disciplinary approach under a new contract.

Other consultants, however, worked in teams within general clinical practice but worked alone when undertaking referrals regarding court proceedings under category 2 of their contract. The advantages of working in a team were, not surprisingly, identified as, first, the opportunity to share information and bring together a range of different views (and thus offset any tendency towards

---

[11] One consultant with considerable experience in this field (who was one of five additional child psychiatrists with whom extensive pilot work was undertaken) reported having decided to refuse to undertake any further referrals in public law proceedings because budget cuts had resulted in the loss of a multi-disciplinary approach in her unit.

over-identification with one party) and, second, the opportunity to obtain the right specialist for particular tasks within the overall family assessment (e.g. adding the skills of a clinical or educational psychologist). The disadvantages of working in a multi-disciplinary team, however, were the tensions that could arise, partly because local authority legal services departments always wanted the consultant psychiatrist to write the report and if necessary appear in court, whether or not he or she agreed that this was what was clinically necessary.[12]

## *Ethical dilemmas: doctor to the family* and *an adviser to the court?*

Given the contexts in which most of these consultants undertook work for public law proceedings (i.e. privately or under category 2 work), it is not surprising to find that most instructions accepted by them in the 12 months before the interviews were in fact for new cases, that is, cases in which the consultant had no previous or ongoing clinical commitment to children and parents. However, consultants raised concerns about the ethical issues that arose for them when they had treated or were currently undertaking work with a child and parents, and where they were asked to move to a forensic exercise within legal proceedings. These concerns arose whether or not the request came in the context of a piece of work that would fall within contracted work for a local authority or whether such work would be undertaken under category 2. For example:

> "I actually find it increasingly difficult and I'm only really beginning to understand this the more I get involved. I'm finding it increasingly difficult to work with two commitments, clinician to the family and expert to the court. I've done it two or three times [and] it makes me feel very uncomfortable ... so I prefer dealing with families that are new to me ... I do occasionally appear as an expert witness in ongoing clinical cases but, generally speaking, I prefer not to." (L8)

> "You need to be clear. You can't undertake something as treatment and then turn it into a forensic report, *without saying to the family, 'Is this okay?'* [emphasis added]. I can think of several cases where we've had long-term involvement with a family and then somebody comes along and says give us a forensic report on this family and I say, 'Not until I've got the family's consent, no'. And sometimes the

---

[12] There are some attempts through training initiatives to shift advocates' and parties' preference for a consultant every time – see Chapter 6.

family understandably say no. And then I say to the local authority: 'No way ... '." (N12)

Moreover, consultants said that simply explaining the change of role to parents (or children) does not necessarily facilitate the switch in 'mindset' that they are expected to make from doctor to the family, to agent/adviser to the court. Consultants felt this issue was seldom addressed or fully understood by courts or other professionals.

The question of whether clinicians *should* accept instructions in public law cases where they have a prior therapeutic commitment to a child and parent is not a new problem. It could equally have occurred in referrals for expert assessments in proceedings before the Children Act 1989.[13] However, following the Children Act, because of the substantial increase in referrals to experts by local authorities and because, after the Cleveland inquiry, all professionals are concerned to protect children from multiple examinations by different experts, this issue takes on new significance.

Guardians addressing this situation have argued that there are both advantages and disadvantages to staying with a clinician who has an established clinical responsibility for a child and family. However, experiences of retaining the same clinician for care proceedings have led some guardians to argue that the disadvantages are beginning to outweigh the perceived benefits. For example, staying with a clinician already instructed by a local authority can present case management problems for guardians – partly because some parents will not see such an expert as truly independent and thus may be more likely to contest a subsequent report (Brophy & Bates, 1999).

Thus, the ethical and practical concerns posed by clinicians must be added to the problems for parents (of a breakdown of trust and confidence in a clinician) and the case management problems raised for guardians. Guardians are concerned to protect children from multiple examinations, keep delays in cases to a minimum but also to maintain the active participation of parents in proceedings – not least because of the implications for children regarding possible future contact and any prospects for reunification of children and parents. Guardians argued that if parents 'throw in the towel' because they feel all the professionals are united against them and their doctor may well betray their trust, then in practice proceedings may do very little to

---

[13] Although it appears that before the Children Act consultants producing reports after referrals via this route were mostly referred to as 'professional witnesses'. There was some blurring of the distinction, the implications of which are discussed in the final chapter.

meet certain principles underscoring the Children Act, for example those aimed at ensuring increased parental participation, encouraging contact between parents and children, and returning children to their parents where this is practical (Brophy & Bates, 1999).

## *Numbers of cases, numbers of appointments and length of experience in clinical and legal arenas*

Consultants confirmed that referrals in public law proceedings are continuing to rise.[14] Estimates for the number of public law cases undertaken in the 12 months before the interviews varied considerably, from 2 to 100, with the national experts tending to undertake more cases per year than local experts.[15] As an estimated proportion of total case-load, the range for national experts was between 10% and 100% (100% for the consultant retired from NHS practice and only undertaking this type of work privately; 80% for the consultant who was semi-retired from the NHS). For local experts, however, the range was much smaller, 2–50% of total case-load, but for half this group the estimated proportion of court work to total clinical case-load was 12% or less. These figures were based on consultants' estimates and, in the absence of supporting material,[16] further research in this field is likely to be necessary. But, given the enormous complexity of many cases, some of these estimates may cause some concern: a total of 75–100 cases per year would be more than one case per week.

The number of times a family may be seen during the course of a clinical assessment can vary, depending of course on the complexity of a case but also on the personal practices of individual consultants. For example, clinicians may decide it is their responsibility to see a family after the assessment, to go over the report and opinion and to make it clear to the parents what changes they would have to make in order for that opinion to change. This study highlighted some variations in working practices and this issue requires more detailed

---

[14] Only one consultant felt there had been a decrease in referrals over the past 12 months.

[15] The national consultants each estimated they were undertaking 12, 15, 50, 50–75 and 100 cases per year (data missing for one participant), the 'local' consultants 2, 9, 9, 10, 10, 12, 25, 50, 65/66 and 100 cases per year (data missing for one participant).

[16] For various reasons, which included the likelihood of increasing the refusal rates in the study, consultants were not asked to do any preparatory work for interviews or to produce any paperwork.

TABLE 3
*Assessments for public law proceedings:*
*number of likely appointments with a child psychiatrist*

| 1 | Up to 2 | Up to 3 | Up to 4 | Up to 5 | 6+ |
|---|---|---|---|---|---|
| N4 | – | N16 | L6 | L14 | L2 |
| N5 | – | N17 | – | – | L3 |
| N12 | – | L8 | – | – | L7 |
| N18 | – | L10 | – | – | L9 |
| L15 | – | – | – | – | L13<br>L19 |

research because there are indications that the number of appointments child psychiatrists undertake may be closely linked to the employment or contractual basis under which this work is accepted. Table 3 indicates that the national experts tended to see families only once, on one afternoon, partly due to the distances they had to travel. All the consultants seeing families just once were working privately, or accepting instructions under category 2 work. Consultants who tended to see families for six or more appointments tended to be consultants working in local services. Some were taking instructions as category 2 work, while others were accepting instructions from a local authority as part of their NHS commitment.

The experts in this study were all very experienced clinicians. Tables 4 and 5 demonstrates that the minimum number of years at consultant status was four and the maximum was 32, the mean value being 16 years. Moreover, all experts except one had been a consultant for more than five years, which indicates that almost all the respondents had

TABLE 4
*Experts working nationally: number of years as a consultant psychiatrist*
*by number of years as an expert witness (n = 6)*

| Accepting instructions nationally | Number of years as a consultant | Number of years as an expert witness |
|---|---|---|
| N4 | 30 | 12 |
| N5 | 17 | 19 |
| N12 | 16 | 10 |
| N16 | 20 | 10 |
| N17 | 14 | 11 |
| N18 | 32 | 32 |

TABLE 5
*Experts working locally: number of years as a consultant psychiatrist
by number of years as an expert witness (n = 11)*

| Accepting instructions locally | Number of years as a consultant | Number of years as an expert witness |
| --- | --- | --- |
| L2 | 4 | 6 |
| L3 | 18 | 25 |
| L6 | 23 | 10 |
| L7 | 8 | 4 |
| L8 | 9 | 4 |
| L9 | 19 | 4 |
| L10 | 9 | 8 |
| L13 | 14 | 14 |
| L14 | 18 | 21 |
| L15 | 26 | 28 |
| L19 | 14 | 16 |

been consultants before the implementation of the 1989 Children Act in October 1991.

Tables 4 and 5 demonstrate that the majority of consultants interviewed had had experience as an expert witness both before and after the implementation of the Children Act. Six consultants (one national, five local) started taking instructions as an expert witness before they became consultants. This is likely to have been during their senior registrar training under the supervision of a consultant.

Almost all consultants had experience at all levels of the family justice system, that is, in the magistrates' family proceedings court, in a care centre/the Principal Registry and the Family Division of the High Court. All consultants working on a national basis had experience at all levels and those who restricted their work to local referrals were only slightly less likely to have gained experience in the High Court – eight of the 11 such clinicians had some experience in that court.

## Conclusions

The study suggests that the involvement of child psychiatrists in assessments and reports within public law proceedings continues to be achieved largely outside of their mainstream duties and responsibilities within the NHS. It has been a matter of absolute choice among consultants as to whether they undertook this type of work. Moreover, although there are no reliable statistical data on the number of the profession who are both able and willing to undertake this work, all existing evidence indicates that they constitute a very small number of consultants from an already very small subgroup of specialists within psychiatry as a whole.[17]

In the context of reforms to civil litigation concerning children and the introduction of an internal market in the NHS at the beginning of the 1990s, the needs of parties and courts for expert evidence and the responsibilities of CAMHS were not formally reviewed. Evidence indicates that a service for proceedings continued on a largely ad hoc basis and was a matter of personal choice. Indeed, without the dedication of a very small group of committed consultants willing and able to undertake at least some of this work in the evenings and weekends, it is likely the 'system' on which family courts are now so heavily dependent would collapse.

This is not to deny the considerable monetary gains for consultants undertaking this work, or that it is likely to enhance their careers, or that such consultants do not consider such work important. That personal commitment, however, does not negate the need to question whether such an ad hoc response to the provision of a service is good enough. Indeed, it begs a number of questions about whether, in an era of child protection and family support where policy is so clearly driven by notions of partnership, and multi-disciplinary, multi-agency approaches, such a crucial input should continue to rely on the personal choice of a relatively small, albeit highly committed group of clinicians. This approach to need is especially worrying in a system where it appears much work nationally is likely to be undertaken outside of the NHS and is therefore largely unregulated and unaccountable – at least in terms of any medical audit – and where the process offers little formal feedback to clinicians. Moreover, because of the limited numbers of participating clinicians, relationships between courts and particular experts are susceptible to criticism because they may appear rather too cosy.

---

[17] The author is grateful to the Royal College of Psychiatrists for assistance with a statistical survey of members undertaken in the context of further research in this field funded by the Nuffield Foundation. This survey provided the numbers of child and adolescent psychiatrists registered with the Royal College, along with ethnic group status – see note 5, Chapter 1, and Brophy (2000*b*).

# 3 The bearers of gifts? What do child psychiatrists consider they bring to child care proceedings?

## Introduction

It is often suggested that, in this field, it is reputation and court performance that largely determine which particular expert should be appointed, and research lends *some* support to that view.[1] Thus, issues of 'status' and getting a 'heavyweight' or at least an expert whom the judges are said to like are important. This chapter explores the other side of the coin: the contributions that experts themselves consider they bring to cases. Thus, the types of cases referred to child psychiatrists are explored along with the range of questions commonly put to them. In the light of ongoing concerns about the use of skills and expertise over and above that of social work, the study also explored consultants' views and perceptions of their 'added value' to proceedings.

## Presenting problems

In discussing what might be termed the 'presenting problem' or 'the causes of concern' in cases referred to consultants, it is important to

---

[1] For guardians at least, the tried and tested expert is preferred and this includes the expert who is good in court and able to withstand cross-examination (Brophy *et al*, 1999*b*, table 3.2).

begin by specifying the different language and terminology used by professionals in this exercise. Although, *on the whole*, consultants were familiar with the terminology utilised in the child protection arena generally and with the concepts in the Children Act 1989, they did not initially describe their tasks in these terms. Rather, they constructed a narrative (the terms and structure of which were drawn from a wide range of theoretical perspectives and frameworks – see 'Underpinning theoretical perspectives and techniques', below) that represented, in part, the focus of the clinical interview and its findings. This was then 'translated' to meet the questions posed by letters of instruction.[2]

First, a number of consultants specified areas of special clinical or research interest (e.g. emotional abuse, trauma, rehabilitation of children, very young parents, depressed mothers) for which they might be known. A small number identified areas where they would not accept letters of instruction from advocates. For example, one consultant would not accept instructions that concerned allegations of child sexual abuse because she perceived this as an area that required very specialist skills and experience. But most consultants did not describe their cases according to the categories used to register children on the Child Protection Register (i.e. physical injury, sexual abuse, emotional abuse, neglect). Some stressed that they focused on all areas concerned with the care and development of children and adolescents. One consultant, for example, described himself as "a bog standard psychiatrist". Most consultants, however, were in agreement that whatever the construction of the 'presenting problem' by parties involved in litigation, in practice cases were hardly ever limited to just one area of concern. For example, clinicians argued that physical or sexual abuse of children was usually accompanied by emotional abuse. In practice, whatever consultants were asked to address in letters of instruction, they considered their clinical independence and their medical duty of care to the child demanded a holistic approach to the assessment of children and parents.

---

[2] It is not intended here to debate the detail of this exercise and its implications for the notion of 'competing discourses' (see the Introduction and, for example, King, 1990), but it is important to note that this 'translation' (if that is indeed what takes place), or at least the first step in that procedure, is undertaken by the experts themselves. It is in part directed by the specific questions set by a letter of instruction, but it can also result from the clinicians' own views and opinions as to their role and task. The evidence indicates that this exercise can be part of a dialogue in which the experts are able to reframe the questions posed, and can if necessary seek further directions from the court for this exercise.

# What do parties generally want from child psychiatrists?

Overall, there were a number of issues on which consultants were likely to comment – whether or not they were requested to do so in a letter of instruction. So, for example, most were usually asked and would comment on whether a child has suffered or is suffering what amounted to significant harm, on the risks to the child and on the parent's ability, willingness and capacity to change. Commenting on whether or not a child was suffering significant harm was often described by consultants as almost always their job, but whether that was an additional activity to one already undertaken by other professionals in a case is less clear. For example, some experts argued that they were not always asked this question, not because it was irrelevant but because it was often obvious. Indeed, one national expert commented that, in most of the instructions he received, the child's status according to the threshold criteria was seldom in doubt. That was not therefore the central issue he was being asked to address; rather, the focus of concern for professionals was 'Where do we go from here?'

In breaking down the required tasks, the question of whether a child was *at risk* of suffering significant harm was seen as a central feature in the assessment exercise. As most consultants stated: "Yes that would nearly always be the case … a definite part of my task"; "The local authority are always interested in this one"; "Yes, that's much more in my area because we're looking at what's happened and what is likely to happen". In this context (of what is likely to happen) almost all consultants were asked to comment on a parent's ability to change. Only two consultants said this was not routinely asked. While it may not always be an explicit or well-articulated question in letters of instruction, it is seen as part of the package that consultants perceived they should supply. For example, consultants stated: "It's something that's always expected of me, but it's not always asked"; "No, you're not always asked, but implicitly you are"; "Yes, that's usually what you are being asked, really".

The Children Act 1989 placed a specific duty on local authorities to work towards returning children to their parents unless that was considered inconsistent with the child's welfare.[3] Half the sample stated they were always asked to comment on prospects for re-unification:

---

[3] Section 23(6), which underpins the general duty under section 17 to promote the upbringing of children by their families.

"Yes, that's a particular area where I think solicitors know I will be able to make a contribution." (L7)

But even if consultants were not asked to address this issue, most said they would comment on it anyway, for example:

"I don't think I am always asked this ... but it's something I would very frequently put in my report." (L19)

The question of which court order might be most appropriate and what contact and placement arrangements should be made for a child frequently depend on the assessment and recommendations of experts in the field of child and family psychiatry (Bates & Brophy, 1996). Whether in principle these are appropriate issues for child psychiatrists to address directly is debatable – at least according to some guardians (Brophy & Bates, 1999). Most consultants were not routinely asked to comment on the type of order appropriate in a particular case – but almost half said they would comment on this issue anyway. Some consultants thought this issue was outside their remit – but they might nevertheless offer an opinion:

"That's changed a bit actually. I used to think that was not the job of a child psychiatrist ... and I still think that it probably isn't ... but, certainly, we do comment on that – I do comment." (L13)

"I have come more and more to the view that I should give a view on this, but I think the expert isn't crucially expected to." (N16)

Despite contemporary debates about the importance of contact between children and their birth parents,[4] surprisingly, not all consultants in this sample were routinely asked to comment on the issue of future contact, but there were clear divergences of views about the role of the expert with regard to the question of contact. For example, some consultants felt that questions about contact were now

---

[4] During the 1980s, a growing body of research argued that when children are separated from their families their well-being is enhanced if they maintain links with their family and friends. Maintaining links is also seen as an important ingredient in ensuring that children can leave accommodation or care and return to families and friends (and the majority of children – some 80% – do so). It has also been argued that contact can be important for children who may never return home, because they function better psychologically, socially and educationally and develop a better sense of identity if they are able to maintain links with and hold a realistic picture of their family (e.g. Millham *et al*, 1986; Thoburn, 1994). The Department of Health (1989, principles 5, 15 and 16; 1991, para. 6.9) stresses the importance of contact.

part of the 'package' routinely expected from them and some would comment on this issue whether or not it was included in the instructions. One expert, however, felt the importance of contact had been "oversold" to the legal arena. He, like others (e.g. Hester & Radford, 1996) argued that the literature in this field was in fact rather poor, and that social workers and courts have tended to take a blanket approach, "hammering away at it in every case". Professionals, he argued, have become insufficiently critical or open to the view that contact with a parent or parents may not always be in a child's interests.[5]

Most experts would nevertheless make recommendations about contact in their report, although this tended to be on the principle of whether contact was appropriate for a child rather than the detail of arrangements. Indeed, this latter task was sometimes seen as somewhat tedious and better left to the social worker and guardian to work out.

Consultants were also asked whether, under the new regime of much more specificity in letters of instruction, they were given sufficient space/flexibility to comment on "any other aspects of a case". In view of some of the responses to earlier questions, in which consultants stated that there were issues on which they would comment whether or not they were asked to do so, one might think this question somewhat irrelevant, since clearly most consultants do not feel constrained by any boundaries set by letters of instruction. However, since consultants reported that most letters of instruction continued to carry this final open-ended request as a semi-permanent fixture, the majority did not perceive directions aimed at achieving greater specificity within letters instruction[6] as a limitation on the role of the expert witness. And a few consultants saw letters of instruction as totally negotiable:

> "I may take no notice of the questions because I'll say what I think best for the child." (L5)

> "and I will add my own questions if necessary" (L8)

Most consultants were not routinely asked to comment on children's wishes and feelings, but a majority reported that they would comment on this aspect even though not specifically instructed to do so. Most consultants also reported being unlikely to be asked to address the relevance of age, gender, 'race', culture, ethnicity or religious

---

[5] And research and practices in cases of domestic violence increasingly support this view: see, for example, Hester & Radford (1996) and Newham Social Services (1999). The issue of contact between children and violent parents has subsequently been taken forward by the Advisory Board on Family Law, Children Act Sub-Committee (1999*a*,*b*).

[6] For example, *Re G (Minors) (Expert Witnesses)* [1994] 2 FLR 291.

persuasion for a child. They were also unlikely to comment upon these issues unless they themselves identified a specific issue relevant to a case.

## Ethical dilemmas: making recommendations as to children's future therapeutic needs

Most experts reported that they were always asked to comment on a child's therapeutic needs; even where they were not requested to do so, most would nevertheless comment on this issue in their report. When it came to making specific recommendations, however, this raised substantial dilemmas, largely because of the national shortage of CAMHS and thus the likelihood of local services being able to take recommendations forward. This resource problem resulted in a variety of practices with regard to quite where to pitch treatment recommendations in reports. The ethical and practical dilemmas and the resultant practices are discussed in Chapter 5.

## The risk assessment – a multi-professional exercise

All consultants interviewed were undertaking risk assessments of parents or carers, and all saw that task as part of their responsibility and remit: it was part of the package expected of child psychiatrists. However, they were not the only discipline with responsibility for that exercise and this was seen as an important clinical point for professionals in the family justice system to understand. Adult psychiatrists, forensic psychiatrists and social workers were also seen as having a role in the assessment of risk and, this was not necessarily seen as duplication. For example:

> "I think we can do parenting risk assessments; I think we are quite good at that, but when it involves adult psychiatric illness, I think we could be shot down in court ... because we're not adult psychiatrists." (N4)

But boundaries could be transgressed and it was not just courts that could get it wrong:

> "My current *bête noire* is about the difference ... between adult and child psychiatrists, and I feel very strongly that some adult psychiatrists aren't trained to assist children in their needs ... it's extremely important that instructions to adult psychiatrists are very focused on diagnosis, treatment required, prognosis, sort of likely effects of the illness on their parenting availability, but not actually

on them as a parent. Whereas adult psychiatrists often stray a bit into commenting on parenting more generally and they're often asked to, and I feel they would do themselves a better service if they stuck more tightly to the issues." (L2)

Child psychiatrists argued that social workers have to know what the risks are, need to be able to identify risks and potential risks, and should comment on them, but, to quote one consultant:

> "I think the child psychiatrist's there to turn a social worker's worries about poor attachment into a reasonably reliable account of what the attachment is like and what effect that's having on the child and what the likely effect will be." (L2)

In effect, *one* of the tasks of the child psychiatrist was to validate the information and the risk assessments done by others. And the family justice system, in drawing on clinical expertise for this work, must also take on board the clinical principle that risk assessments should rarely be undertaken by one person working alone.[7] However, consultants argued that putting together the various aspects of a risk assessment was their responsibility:

> "You can ask adult psychiatrists to do some bits for you, but you still have to revamp it ... so the risk assessment is important but probably needs quite a few people doing it." (L3)

Most experts also stated that a risk assessment is not a certain exercise.[8] It was, in practice, a difficult balancing act, where past harms may be viewed as indicators of future risks. But the balancing act itself was often a source of conflict in care proceedings. Some consultants thought that conflict between experts was often about how certain issues were weighted and thus the degree of risk a parent was judged to represent. But it was this responsibility for putting together a picture for the court that the child psychiatrists argued constituted their particular contribution. In effect, consultants argued they took the risk assessment of others, for example an adult psychiatrist, along with any views about whether a parent was amenable to or responding to treatment, and assessed the implications for parenting in the context

---

[7] This position forms part of the general principles for practice proposed by the Royal College of Psychiatrists' Special Working Party on Clinical Assessment and Management of Risk (1996).

[8] The general principles state: "Risk cannot be eliminated; it can be rigorously assessed and managed, but outcomes cannot be guaranteed" (Royal College of Psychiatrists' Special Working Party on Clinical Assessment and Management of Risk, 1996).

of the particular child. In other words, while the issue of adult mental health remains the territory of the adult psychiatrist, the implications of adult mental health for the parenting of a specific child are clearly the remit of the child psychiatrist.

## Social work assessments

Most consultants were familiar with the comprehensive social work assessment.[9] However, consultants' experiences with regard to the completion of this assessment prior to the instigation of legal proceedings appeared somewhat patchy – they estimated that in about half of all cases referred to them such assessments had not been undertaken before referral.[10]

Where social work assessments had been completed, their quality was seen to vary considerably. Much depended on the skills and experience of the individual social worker and the particular locality. For example:

> "They vary enormously; some of them lighten my load enormously, others are awful." (N4)

> "In this area they are very, very poor." (L2)

> "I have a thing about the yellow or orange book, I mean, there are so many assessment things, I mean, it's almost valueless. It's badly written about families that don't exist ... I think some social workers are stunningly good and conscientious, but sometimes they just get a complete thing in their heads and go charging off in the wrong direction." (L6)

This is not to suggest that consultants thought that social workers did not have a specific contribution to make in complex cases.

---

[9] The Department of Health's (1988) *Protecting Children* was often referred to by practitioners as the 'orange book' for assessment. This guide has been replaced by *Framework for the Assessment of Children in Need and Their Families* (Department of Health *et al*, 2000*a*).

[10] There are of course several reasons why assessments may not have been undertaken by social workers before proceedings: lack of resources or skills in a local authority and lack of parental cooperation are perhaps two major reasons. In one study, 62% of cases included "lack of cooperation with the local authority" as one of a range of reasons for legal proceedings (Bates & Brophy, 1996, table 13). Also, a high staff turnover in many social services departments weakens the ability of local authorities to offer consistency of practice in this field. In addition, a minority of cases may result from emergency procedures (under section 44 of the Children Act 1989) where it has been necessary for a local authority to seek an emergency protection order before the instigation of any assessments.

Consultants expected social workers to examine practical issues, for example parenting skills, rehousing, social networks and support for parents – skills that consultants readily acknowledged they did not have. Indeed, a point often raised by guardians was that child psychiatrists were not generally aware of the social and economic deprivation of most families who are involved in care proceedings and of the links between social class and the likelihood of entry into the care system.[11]

Consultants also thought that social workers had a particular strength in that they usually had the benefit of assessing parents over a period of time: they were less dependent on the snapshot approach that many of these consultants undertook. Some consultants reported some very skilled work from social workers and some very sophisticated reports; in some locations consultants believed that social work assessments were becoming much more organised. But some consultants based in local services also felt that shrinking budgets and lack of resources in social services departments, coupled with the tensions and stresses on social workers, were having a disabling effect on social work practices generally.

There were also particular concerns. Vital information could be missing from social work assessments,[12] the quality of observational work was said to be variable in some areas, some social workers were said to be very process oriented (i.e. lacking in analytical skills) and assessments could lack sufficient information on the interactive nature of a family. Additionally, consultants expressed concern about certain social workers' use and knowledge of theories: they were often fragmented and oversimplified. Consultants reported that bits of theories appeared in social work reports; for example, the notion that it is best for children to be in their own families was indiscriminately applied in cases. Notions of attachment were used by some social workers in ways that concerned consultants; to quote one psychiatrist's experience, the way in which attachment was addressed "indicated they hadn't a clue about attachment theory".[13]

Table 6 shows the issues consultants would like to see included in social work assessments in the cases referred to them. Comparisons

---

[11] Research has outlined the effect of social and economic variables on the likelihood of reception into care (e.g. Bebbington & Miles, 1989), but this does not of course mean that there is a causal link between poverty and child abuse.
[12] For example, one consultant reported that, in a case referred to him, the fact that a child had been hit around the head and suffered two fractures was not included in the documentation.
[13] It should also be noted that one local consultant acknowledged not knowing much about what should be covered in a social work assessment. Also, similar

TABLE 6
*The contents of social work assessments: information required by child psychiatrists and its recommended inclusion in Department of Health guidance*

| Information required by child psychiatrists | Recommended for inclusion by the Department of Health (1988) |
|---|---|
| History of parent's background | Yes |
| Family history, including extended family and genogram | Yes |
| Family functioning | Yes |
| Parents' current relationship | Yes |
| Aspects/quality of parenting | Yes |
| How the child has been functioning | Yes |
| What the child is like (i.e. observations/description of child) | Yes |
| Child's wishes and feelings, individual needs | No |
| A chronology of what has happened so far | Yes |
| What has been tried with family | No |
| A clear account of the concerns | Yes |
| A care plan | Yes |

undertaken with the Department of Health (1988) guidance for social workers that was relevant at the time of the interviews indicated that, in theory at least, most of these issues should be addressed in a comprehensive social work assessment.

There are, however, two areas consultants would like to see addressed by social workers that were not covered in the relevant guidance:

(a) children's wishes and feelings,
(b) what has been tried to date with the child/family.

This discrepancy is probably related to the different uses intended for guidance at the time and the fact that publication (1988) predated the Children Act and the considerable increase in the use of experts to undertake family assessments. Moreover, the Department of Health's guidance (what was the 'orange book' assessment) also included three additional areas for social work assessments that consultants did not mention in any great depth:

(a) finance and physical environment;

---

criticisms of oversimplification and partial views and a failure to consider relevant research have been levelled at some child psychiatrists by guardians. This type of criticism levelled at members of both groups about what constitutes an appropriate level of skill, training and experience and its implications for future policy in this field is considered in the conclusion to this chapter.

  (b) parents' ability to change (arguably this might be included in information of what has already been tried with the family);
  (c) whether parents accept responsibility or at least culpability for the alleged abuse.

Where 'best practice' happens with regard to social work assessments, this exercise has *some* features in common with the work undertaken by child psychiatrists. However, in a legal culture that has been dominated by criticisms about the use of experts, and where the question 'Is all this expert evidence really necessary?' continues to govern almost any discussion in this field, it is important to move beyond the identification of areas of communality and complementary practice. In order to move this debate beyond anecdotal evidence[14] it is necessary to begin by examining how professionals themselves perceive and identify certain professional boundaries of expertise in the assessment of families and what might be termed their specific 'added value'.

## 'Added value': what do child psychiatrists consider they bring to the task of assessing families that is different from that of a social worker?

The narrative from this section of the interviews with consultants is worthy of a book in its own right, and Box 2 does not do full justice to some of the discussion, reasoning and reflective thinking that most

---

**Box 2**
*Training, skills and knowledge: the 'added value' of the child psychiatrist*

- Medical training (and an understanding of how ill health impinges upon functioning and behaviour).
- Training in adult mental illness.
- Training in child mental health.
- Knowledge of the availability and effectiveness of various treatment approaches.
- Training and experience to make a prognosis regarding risks to a child.
- Training in abnormal behaviour of children.
- Research knowledge and experience.
- Substantial experience working with disturbed children and families.
- Additional training in psychology, psychotherapy and family therapy.
- An ability to take a good family history.

---

[14] For example, a view from some social workers and guardians was that child psychiatrists often "don't tell us anything we don't already know".

consultants entered into in answering this question. However, analysis of this material begins to bring us nearer to a model – at least from the perspective of experts themselves – of what might be termed 'added value', in the field of psychiatric family assessments.

Extensive training underscored much of the interviewees' discussion about differences in approaches to family assessments between social workers and psychiatrists:[15]

> "The main thing I'm bringing is a developmental background and some knowledge of the role of the research literature, developmental theories, developmental findings, knowledge of the scope of therapeutic interventions when compared with other sorts of tactical support processes, a more straight psychiatric assessment of parent's mental state and personality function." (L7)

> "It's a much broader training ... you have a grounding in medicine and how ill health can impinge on functioning and behaviour and things ... I'd know about mental health and mental illness and about various treatments for that and the prognosis for that ... the minutiae of child development, physical, mental, emotional ... and some family therapy training ... mental health in the child ... odd behaviours in children ... I have seen thousands of children." (L9)

> "That's a difficult question, isn't it? Well, first of all, our medical background – I think we can often spot things that have been missed ... our psychiatric training; secondly ... we know about adult mental health and that's really important when we are looking at parental functioning and ... our child psychiatric training, which enables us to make psychiatric diagnoses and to know the available treatments, their effectiveness and so on ... also taking histories – I find that social workers aren't very good at taking a proper history ... so taking a history, making observations and being able to separate those two. It's being able to separate observations and understand their relevance in the context of the history – it's not purely psychiatric ... and then of course having a knowledge of the body of research ... and being able to evaluate other people's research and the value of it ... one has knowledge of normal child development and therefore one is far more able to observe deviations from that norm." (N4)

---

[15] The minimum period required in training is defined by the training programmes stipulated by the Royal Colleges (Allen, 1988, pp. 6–7). At the time of this study, doctors were not regarded as trained until they reached consultant status; for child psychiatrists this was generally a minimum of seven years after qualification. As indicated above, the consultants in this sample averaged 16 years at consultant level. A review and rationalisation of medical training is proposed (Department of Health, 2000). Some of the implications of these proposals for future court work are discussed in Chapter 6.

But consultants acknowledged that in many cases referred to them in child protection litigation they would not be making a diagnosis of mental illness as such:

> "being asked for your 'psychiatric opinion' isn't very helpful, and in the majority of cases I get involved in, there isn't a psychiatric diagnosis to be made ... it's about child development and family and social influences on it ... the complexities of those influences on the child's predicament ... assessment of the capacity to change and confidence in doing that." (L14)

A few consultants went on to compare their background and training with that undertaken by social workers. For example:

> "I've three 'A's at A' level ... an MRCPsych ... a DCHGPM, a ... I mean, I've had masses and masses of training, I finished my exams at 32, and I've got a psychology degree and a medical degree and I've got a diploma in child health and mental health and I've got experience in adult clinics and child clinics and psychiatric clinics and it's 25 years' worth of clinical work ... and social workers are coming with a two-year CQSW and one year's training ... I mean, you don't get into medical school with a couple of 'O' levels, which is what can get you onto a CQSW – I mean, it's the intellectual capacity, isn't it?" (L3)

In addition, some consultants acknowledged that, unlike social workers, they were not charged with statutory duties towards children deemed to be at risk. That lack of statutory obligation, undeniably coupled with the power and status accorded consultants, was often experienced as very freeing. For example, consultants interestingly argued they could go more slowly[16] and worry less than people working under a statutory obligation.

What emerges from these discussions is not the importance of medical and psychiatric training *per se*, but rather the range of training and experience child psychiatrists undertake and, in their view at least, the ability to *analyse and synthesise* wide-ranging information. This means bringing together a biological, a social and a psychological perspective. This is coupled with an ability to take case histories, to examine contemporary behaviours in the light of that history, and to form an opinion about what those components might indicate for future parenting possibilities given the immediate and longer-term needs of the child.

---

[16] It is interesting that pressures set by court timetables did not impinge on this discussion, perhaps because this exercise is seen within a clinical rather than a legal framework.

In undertaking such work, *some* of what consultants argued they do is similar to that addressed by social workers. But it is the synthesis of this information, coupled with a clinical opinion of the implications of that information for future parenting possibilities, that differentiates these family assessments from those undertaken by social workers. This is an exercise for which most social workers were seen as neither equipped nor trained.

## Underpinning theoretical perspectives and techniques

Given the wide range of training indicated above, it may not be surprising that questions about the theoretical perspectives, frameworks and techniques employed in assessments for court proceedings produced some thoughtful moments in interviews. In terms of theoretical underpinnings – at least with regard to assessments within litigation – most of these consultants are best described as eclectic in orientation. Psychodynamic theory was most popular, with family systems approaches and techniques providing much of the framework for assessments. But clinicians were seldom wedded to one theoretical perspective for this work. Most were drawing on at least two theoretical approaches and a range of techniques, including attachment and developmental theories (both cognitive and analytic), psychoanalytic and behavioural perspectives and psychotherapeutic techniques.

There was some difficulty in pinning consultants down in this respect, especially, for example, where it appeared they were using approaches that, in principle, are built on very different models of human behaviour, motivation, and views about conscious and unconscious processes and thus the capacity for change in thinking and behaviour. This was not an easy area for clinicians to address and it is doubtful whether they had ever previously been asked to explain how their work for this *particular* field is underscored and theoretically driven. For example, one consultant responded:

> "I don't think I can answer that. I just go and talk to the kids ... I'm not being modest ... I think it's really quality work that I do ... I don't think anybody could do it, because I think its actually quite subtle, but I don't have a technique." (L6)

Asked whether there were any theoretical perspectives or models of human behaviour guiding thinking in relation to this work, this consultant, like others in this sample, initially found it hard to move beyond describing his approach as eclectic. Like many other professionals working in the field of child welfare, being asked to articulate the obvious and unpack taken-for-granted approaches to everyday decision making was not, initially, an easy exercise. But taking the process in a series of stages, looking at parents' experiences of their own parenting, questioning them to get an indication of how much understanding they have of how a child has been affected by events, and eliciting children's worries, concerns and preoccupations were seen as involving a range of theories and techniques.

One consultant's inventory of techniques started with the clinical interview and clinical skills, and included observation of behaviour and inferences from, for example, the use of dolls by children, observation of interaction between children and parents and *sometimes* the use of standardised psychometric tests and questionnaires, for example IQ tests and attainment tests. Table 7 gives an example of one format for the clinical interview used by a consultant working in a major teaching hospital in London.

TABLE 7
*The clinical interview – issues and content*

| Issues | Content |
| --- | --- |
| Reasons for referral | A description and history of main complaint |
| Systematic enquiry | A child's general health, eating, sleeping, urinary/bowl symptoms, physical activity, speech, vision, hearing, tics and mannerisms, attack disorders, antisocial behaviour, sex information or problems, emotional state (e.g. happy, worries, sulks, tempers, fearful) |
| Family history | The mother's and father's backgrounds and own parenting, siblings, education, employment, marriages, health and illness and treatments, personality, child-rearing practices and discipline, home environment, finances and other family history, including physical, psychiatric and learning difficulties |
| Developmental history | For example, conception, pregnancy, delivery, neonatal conditions, mother's condition, early feeding and sleeping habits, temperament |
| Developmental milestones | Walking, speech, bowel/bladder control, past illnesses and hospital admissions |
| Separations | Timing and responses to separations |
| Schools and peer relationships | Including preschool experiences |
| Temperamental characteristics and interests | For example, play and hobbies |
| Examination of the child | Formulation and, in general clinical practice, a proposed treatment |

With regard to the theories/models underpinning his work, this same consultant argued:

> "I'm not a psychoanalyst ... but I do use a lot of psychoanalytic insights and ideas. Basically I'm an empiricist. I base my work on research findings plus clinical experience." (N4)

In discussing the techniques and theories they used, some consultants moved between their training and 'presenting problems', drawing on different aspects of their training for different parts of the family assessment exercise. For example:

> "[I'm] using my training as an adult psychiatrist to assess a parent's personality and mental state, I'm using skills based on my knowledge as a child psychiatrist in terms of parenting skills, and psychological models of parenting to assess and probe what they are telling me ... I'm using information from attachment theory ... [and] techniques derived from psychotherapy with children to understand their anxieties, defences, attachments, and then I'm using my family interview techniques, structured family interview techniques to explore boundary issues of control and alliances that affect the family." (N17)

> "I use direct observation of behaviours and relationships. I've got training in strategic family therapy and I use that ... I have individual clinical skills in terms of asking adult psychiatric questions and my cognitive–behavioural training with offenders which I can use ... I've got training in developmental child paediatrics ... I do sometimes go through stuff like the special parenting programme stuff ... life skills work ... I've got things like family assessments, psychological family assessments ... and I can use a whole bank of testing material if I want to."

As to a theoretical perspective underpinning her work, this consultant continued:

> "I think I had a Freudian training and although I don't work in a psychodynamic way I think that really helps ... so there is a kind of Freudian psychodynamic basis to the assessments ... and I think my cognitive–behavioural stuff works very well with people." (L13)

Other consultants, while not totally dismissing certain perspectives in favour of others, nevertheless said their work was more clearly informed by one technique and one perspective:

> "I see them as a 'family' ... we've always done a lot of family work in this team, I did some adult psychotherapy training ... and I did some group training."

With regard to the theoretical underpinnings of assessments for court work, this consultant continued:

> "I've always been more psychotherapeutic, I'm not a behaviourist by nature." (L9)

Some areas were seen as central to the psychiatrist's task:

> "I don't think you can be a psychiatrist ... without [knowing] a lot about psychodynamic theories as an underpinning ... I'm also interested in systemic models in thinking about family behaviour and behavioural techniques." (L10)

Underlying some of these discussions was a recurrent theme, arguably perhaps more applicable to therapeutic practice than assessments for courts, about what 'works' with a family. This was seen as an important starting point. For example, with regard to discussing the techniques employed, one consultant argued he used the whole range of available techniques, drawn from a background and training in a range of theoretical perspectives:

> "I've been through the whole gambit of group work and psycho-therapy and psychoanalysis and family therapy, way before I even started forensic work ... and subsequently in individual psycho-therapy, psychoanalysis and group psychoanalysis in the mid-'60s. ... So, I mean, I've had a whole range of exposures, but I am absolutely certain that in an eclectic approach it is the individual's impact upon the family that counts." (L15)

Thus, although a background in medicine and psychiatric training formed the basis of approaches to assessments for litigation purposes, they were seldom the only skills deployed. Nor, indeed, in the majority of cases were they necessarily seen as the most essential skills: these consultants seldom made a diagnosis of mental illness as such. But early training provided a foundation on which most consultants had built subsequent training and skills in child and family work. As demonstrated above, many of the techniques and theoretical perspec-tives engaged were drawn from models of human behaviour and development that are not essentially medical in origin. In addition to having a foundation in medicine, these professionals were utilising theories and techniques that also form the basis of other disciplines (e.g. clinical psychology, various forms of psychotherapy) and are used by others working with children and parents in the psychotherapeutic field. Indeed, child psychiatrists appear to be drawing heavily on these theories and techniques. In terms of clinical practice, however, they are seldom wedded to one theoretical perspective and one technique.

Rather, they have a range of perspectives and techniques at their disposal and their approach tended to be eclectic.

The term 'eclectic' can be used as something of an escape clause, to obstruct attempts to explore practices or to unpack what is often called 'trained intuition' or simply woolly thinking in this field. It might be argued there is evidence of some ducking and weaving in some of the responses described above – or at least some evidence of muddled thinking. However, most respondents in fact tried very hard to answer these questions. And while these data beg some further research,[17] the study does answer part of the question of why there is a relatively frequent use of child psychiatrists in proceedings: their work and expertise are not limited to issues of child 'mental illness' as such – although indications are that adult mental health issues feature in about one-third of cases involving experts (Brophy *et al*, 1999*b*, table 4.9).

There are also some undeniable strengths in the eclectic approaches identified in this field but consultants did not try to duck the negative connotations attached to the term. What emerged from discussions was that, for these consultants at least, it is that very eclectic practice that separated the work of the child psychiatrist from that of the other professionals assessing children and parents. This ability to draw on a range of clinical training, theories and techniques constituted a further part of their 'added value' – the extra cachet and the distinguishing feature of their particular work in the field of family assessments.

Following the Children Act 1989, the central question most often posed for professionals addressing cases of child abuse and neglect was, in effect, 'Where do we go from here?' Once all the professionals involved considered that the evidence met the threshold criteria, it was this latter exercise that became the most important, but also, at times, the most controversial feature in the overall remit of the child psychiatrist. It is controversial in that the exercise of synthesis, or fusion of multi-dimensional measures, theories, techniques and indeed attitudes, is usually undertaken by one person and may go unchallenged and under-exposed to scientific or peer review. As the clinicians themselves demonstrated, they do not routinely attempt a systematic application of a specific set of principles drawn from one field. Indeed, the strength of their eclectic approach, in clinical practice at least, lies in finding what works for a particular child and family. As a discursive practice, it starts with the particular child and parents. However, where

---

[17] In practice this work provides a basis for further investigations about the relationship between what child psychiatrists say they do and the frameworks on which they rely, and what happens in practice.

this approach forms the basis for court work, the nature of the enterprise itself and the fact that so little of it is open to research or debate in the usual scientific journals have arguably done little to give the outside world or other professionals in the family justice system a better idea of what child psychiatrists consider they have to offer and how their work is underpinned.

It is not the purpose of this book to debate the scientific status of this exercise (see Dawes, 1994), or to look at the assumptions behind assertions in the discourse (e.g. about the construction of the self and individual 'pathology' and the reliability of predictions of clinicians over those of others), or to examine how historically these medical and psychological discourses have informed legal practices. Rather, the aim of this part of the study was to start that exercise by elucidating the discourses through which consultants in the field of child psychiatry described their particular contributions to the questions set by advocates and courts when addressing allegations of child neglect or maltreatment and to the exercise imposed under section 31 of the Children Act 1989 (see Fig. 1, p. 9).

## Assessing children and parents from Black and other ethnic minority households

In view of the relatively high proportion of Black children and children of mixed parentage who appear in care proceedings that involve experts (Brophy *et al*, 1999*b*, table 4.2; Brophy, 2000*a*), consultants were asked whether they thought their conceptual frameworks translated across cultural boundaries and whether they had received any training on the assessment of Black and other ethnic minority families.

Almost half the sample had received some training in this sphere.[18] Some had not had any formal training but said they had informed themselves because their catchment area included Black and other ethnic minority families. Some consultants had experiences of undertaking referrals involving children of mixed parentage and from Black minority groups that had left them with a sense of unease. For example:

> "I have had experience of referrals involving black families and I'm slightly uncomfortable about it because I think they would prefer to have a black psychiatrist, and I think where possible they [the

---

[18] The training mentioned was a study day provided by the Royal College of Psychiatrists, a study day with a legal practitioner in this field, and some training offered by a major teaching hospital in London.

instructing parties] should find them someone who parents find appropriate." (L6)

One consultant had a specific research and clinical interest in issues of 'race', ethnicity and child protection issues and reported being frequently instructed because of this background. But for other experts, partly because their catchment area did not include many Black families, specific training did not appear to have been undertaken.

The question of whether prevailing conceptual frameworks translate across cultural boundaries produced some interesting discussion. For some consultants, there were certain issues that they felt applied to most cultures. Whether parents were able to meet their child's emotional and practical needs and the role of attachment theory as a means of addressing some of these concerns were recurrent themes. For example, one consultant argued:

> "If a child's emotionally damaged in terms of the way they make relationships, now that to my mind, as it were, crosses most racial and cultural backgrounds." (N5)

Some were less happy with the notion that *all* ideas about child development and attachment were cross-cultural:

> "It's clear that what is culturally normal in terms of attachment patterns would obviously be different because children aren't brought up in the same family base." (L2)

This consultant went on to discuss as an example a case that demonstrated the anguish and distress experienced by a refugee child following the loss of an extended family of carers. A further consultant was less than happy with some of the psychological materials available for testing children. This psychiatrist gave an example of a word association test that he said he would not use with Black children. Another psychiatrist was adamant that traditional conceptual frameworks were not necessarily applicable across cultural boundaries; his approach when asked to undertake a cross-cultural assessment would be to find someone else to do it.

A further consultant, interestingly, took some time to reflect on his response to earlier questions and his defence of 'eclecticism' as a description of his theoretical framework and techniques. With regard to whether his framework could be applied across cultural boundaries, he concluded:

> "If I'm eclectic, it shouldn't be, should it ... if you adapt your techniques for each individual ... you take into account the context in which you are seeing them, their culture, background and so

forth … and you deal differently with families from different parts of a community." (L19)

Given the range of responses it seems clear that the role and significance of issues of 'race', culture and ethnicity in the assessment of Black and other ethnic minority families requires further work. One aim should be to identify relevant research and clinical debate and writing in this field[19] but further aims should include exploring ways in which available work can be incorporated into individual and multi-disciplinary training opportunities.[20]

## 'Gilding the lily': using psychiatrists to add status and power

In view of current debates about the misuse of experts, interviews also explored with consultants whether they received requests for assessments that they felt were inappropriate. Over two-thirds said they had, on occasion. But responses did not suggest this was a constant and overwhelming problem and certainly did not indicate that this constituted the majority of their referrals.[21]

Where examples of what might be termed 'rubber stamping' emerged, consultants said local authority legal departments and courts were often the cause of that type of referral. Courts were seen to want 'a doc in the box'; local authority legal services wanted to ensure cases were watertight and a supporting psychiatric opinion was seen as the best guarantee. This type of referral could also, on occasion, emerge from a case where a guardian wanted an expert to support a social work decision that was felt to be borderline.

## More 'added values' from child psychiatrists

In extremely complex and difficult cases where issues become clouded or where proceedings become bogged down, some consultants

---

[19] This issue has been taken forward in research funded by the Nuffield Foundation (see Brophy, 2000*a,b*).
[20] It may also be relevant for instructing parties to ascertain with proposed experts whether they have undertaken any training or have any experience in working cross-culturally before issuing instructions for an assessment of Black or other ethnic minority children and parents.
[21] That is, responses were of the type 'Sometimes', 'Yes I can at times' – in other words, although such referrals can happen, they were not identified as a central problem, at least for these clinicians.

considered they could make a contribution by working with professionals and parents to untangle the issues and move a case forward. It is important to stress in this context that consultants readily acknowledged there were occasions where all professionals – including the expert – were baffled by a case. Clinicians in this sample gave examples of where they had met with both the local authority and the guardian to discuss cases that presented very perplexing features to all concerned.

In attempting to help parties to move a case on, consultants argued that the impact of their work could be identified in the response of parents. For example, following the filing of their report, parents might decide not to continue to contest an order. That was seen as a very positive contribution. Such a decision on the part of parents could result from the report itself, or from a more direct intervention by a consultant. For example, one consultant stated:

> "I've said to parents. 'There's no point in pursuing this you know, you're not going to win, in view of my report you know' – I leant very heavily on one of the parents." (N5)

But interventions could also help change the stance of a local authority:

> "I think I sometimes move parties to a more workable situation and I can sometimes move social services to a workable situation." (L3)

Overall, however, consultants felt their influence at this level was quite variable. Guardians and solicitors could be influenced quite a lot but parents, it seemed, less so. Some psychiatrists also said that, in delivering negative views to parents, they could on occasion make it clear to parents what they would have to achieve in order to change the situation. Some consultants thought there was a value in them undertaking that task as an independent source, with no particular axe to grind. It is also arguably the case that their status as a doctor rather than a social worker has the potential to soften the ultimatum and perhaps make it appear more palatable.

## Conclusions

Sections of the interview that focused on what information consultants generally provided, views about levels of certainty in the risk assessment exercise, views about social work assessments and their own added value and the theories and techniques on which they draw revealed variation and diversity but also consistency and congruity in practices.

There was some variation in the types of cases experts would take on and some experts had particular areas of expertise that were clearly more appropriate to some cases than others. Some experts restricted their referrals to areas of a developing research or clinical interest, while others were willing to work across the range of issues and concerns likely to arise in public law applications. There are, thus, areas of sub-specialisation within the speciality of child psychiatry. That is not surprising. But this finding suggests one reason why some professional parties look to experts outside of their immediate catchment area for assessments. In addition to the general limitations of many local CAMHS in this field, parties may also be looking for very specific skills and expertise for certain cases.

Equally, indications are that, whatever the issue, for the most part instructing parties now seek a complete package of information from child psychiatrists but with a heavy emphasis on questions about the future: the future needs of a child and the future risks that parents represent and their willingness, ability and potential for change. This is not to suggest that borderline cases are not referred to these consultants but, for these consultants at least, the evidence indicates such cases do not constitute the vast majority of their public law case-load. Although most consultants had experiences of being instructed where they felt they were not needed, these cases were not the majority. In other words, for the most part, consultants considered their skills and expertise were appropriately sought.

There was much consistency in views about the complexity and multi-disciplinary nature of the risk assessment exercise. Whatever advocates might want, all consultants argued that this is not a precise science. Risk could not be eliminated: it could be rigorously assessed and managed, but outcomes could not be guaranteed and the assessment itself was seldom one to be undertaken by a single practitioner.

While early case law directed experts to stick to the instructions and much has been done to try to improve the quality and specificity of letters, a few consultants saw letters of instruction as almost entirely negotiable. Subsequent practices have indicated that there should be room for some discussion if experts have concerns about instructions and if necessary they can be discussed and amended. But they are not open to unilateral amendment by the appointed expert.[22] Some consultants routinely recommended a specific court order, whether or not they were asked to do so. Some resisted this move only to be asked by the judge what order he or she would like the judge to make.

---

[22] And experts can expect strong questions in court as to their credibility if they have gone inappropriately beyond instructions.

Bearing in mind the considerable complexity of many cases that involve expert evidence and the likelihood therefore that most cases will be transferred,[23] the range of training and experience in clinical practice articulated by these consultants is, in principle, extensive and impressive. They were also fairly consistent in views about how this extensive training had an added value to proceedings. While they were less consistent in adherence to particular theories and techniques for this work, there was, nevertheless, a degree of congruity of approach, a consensus in that most were not wedded to one framework but were somewhat eclectic, drawing on a range of theoretical frameworks and methods. This eclecticism, however, was a less persuasive approach when it came to discussing assessments of Black and other ethnic minority children and parents. There was a diversity of views about whether preferred frameworks and techniques were equally applicable, but a growing recognition, for some at least, that this was an area of practice that gave rise to some concern.

But there was also some recognition of the diversity of functions that experts could serve, for example in helping parties move forward, working with parents and advocates where outcomes were likely to be unpalatable for parents, and working with professionals to try to clarify issues in highly complex and difficult cases. What was not so heavily emphasised by these consultants, but which has been highlighted elsewhere, is the role that they can play in reviewing existing evidence in a case and advising advocates on the strengths and weaknesses of expert reports already filed, including the questions that might be appropriate should the case come to trial.

---

[23] For example, information from a national random survey of cases revealed about a third of cases included a report from an adult psychiatrist (Brophy *et al*, 1999*b*, table 4.9). Just over half (53%) of cases that contain any expert evidence are likely to be transferred to the care centre or High Court (Brophy *et al*, 1999*b*, table 4.3).

# 4    The new legal agenda:
those 'on the receiving end'

## Introduction

A number of issues stand out in discussions about the use of experts in public law proceedings since the Children Act 1989, but most are rooted in four concerns:

(a) increases in costs and delays in proceedings;
(b) lack of court control over parties' use of experts;
(c) lack of specificity in instructions to experts;
(d) and a lack of clarity about the roles and responsibilities of experts in proceedings.

As outlined in Chapter 1, attention has therefore been focused on:

(a) how courts should exert more control over parties' use of experts (e.g. Booth, 1996; Practice Direction [1995][1]);
(b) improving the quality of letters of instruction to experts;[2]

---

[1] In addressing case management, the President's Practice Direction [1995] Fam Law, 156 stated: "the importance of reducing cost and delay of civil litigation makes it necessary for the court to assert greater control over the preparation for and conduct of hearings than has hitherto been customary ... (2) The court will accordingly, exercise its discretion to limit ... (d) the issues on which it wishes to be addressed ... (3) to confine the issues and evidence called to what is reasonably considered to be essential for the proper presentation of their case; (b) to reduce or eliminate issues for expert evidence". After this study, a further practice direction addressed this issue – see note 14.

[2] For example, *Re M (Minors) (Care Proceedings: Child's Wishes)* [1994] 1 FLR 749; *Re G (Minors) (Expert Witnesses)* [1994] 2 FLR 291.

(c) specifying the boundaries of expertise between the judge and the expert;[3]
(d) outlining the responsibilities and duties of experts.[4]

In addition, where experts disagree in cases, in an effort to reduce the length of a fully contested final hearing and to locate in advance those issues on which the court may have to make a finding of 'fact', experts are now expected to meet before the final hearing and produce a statement of agreement or disagreement.[5]

Many of the changes instigated above have been considered beneficial both to the court and to the expert witness, although arguably the emphasis has been more clearly on attempts to reduce costs and duration of cases and particularly the duration of final hearings.[6] Nevertheless, these changes mark out a new and very different agenda for those child welfare specialists who are both able and willing to work in this field. In this chapter the views and experience of consultants on the receiving end of these changes are explored. Issues such as the writing of reports, approaches to making recommendations and the use of research evidence are explored. In addition, given the hopes for improved practices that underscore these changes, consultants' views about the achievements of care proceedings under the Children Act are also explored.

## 'On the receiving end': letters of instruction after the Act

Since the implementation of the Children Act, a central feature of directions to experts in care proceedings has been the clear statement that an expert's first responsibility is to the court, not the instructing party. The expert's key function is to assist the court in reaching a decision by helping it to understand the case. Thus, whichever party instructs and pays an expert witness, that witness has an overriding duty to the court.

---

[3] For example, *Re S & B (Minors) (Child Abuse: Evidence)* [1990] 2 FLR 489; *Re AB (Child Abuse: Expert Witnesses)* [1995] 1 FLR 181.
[4] *Re R (A Minor) (Expert's Evidence)* [1991] 1 FLR 291n; *Re M (Minors) (Care Proceedings) (Child's Wishes)* [1991] 1 FLR 794n.
[5] *Re C (Expert Evidence: Disclosure)* [1995] 1 FLR 204.
[6] Although there has been increasing recognition that many clinicians are already overstretched and therefore their services should be engaged with care and attempts should be made to ensure they do not, for example, have to waste time in court waiting to be called to give evidence.

Guidance has been issued both to courts and to parties about the need to avoid biased instructions and to increase the specificity of letters of instruction to experts – it is no longer appropriate for parties simply to ask a child psychiatrist for a psychiatric opinion of a family. However, research indicates that, unless parties cannot agree about an application for leave to instruct an expert, courts seldom become involved in decisions about the selection of particular experts or the finer details of instructions and this is especially so in the early stages of a case in the family proceedings court (Brophy & Bates, 1999).

Most of the consultants in this sample received instructions from the local authority, the guardian and, to a lesser extent, the Official Solicitor. With regard to the parties most commonly involved in care proceedings (the local authority, the guardian and the parents), some consultants expressed a very clear preference for instructions from the guardian, because guardians were viewed as having no axe to grind and paid well.[7] Also, the letter of instruction was usually much better: "[guardians] are well trained, they know what they want", "they know how to instruct consultants"[8] and, "they specify the time to be spent on a case". Moreover, when consultants were working on instructions from the guardian, they felt they were seen as more independent, more 'for the child', and it was felt that this position was generally likely to carry more status and more weight in court.

Most of the consultants also undertook instructions from local authorities and here there was some criticism of letters of instruction. Interviews highlighted some of the problems that can result from joint arrangements (i.e. when a health trust and a local authority enter into contracts whereby a clinician supplies a number of assessments and court reports per year). One consultant who was contracted to provide assessments for a local authority reported he was considering stopping this type of arrangement because he was dissatisfied with the referrals. He reported that requests for assessments were sometimes vague and not well thought out. He was also expected to be in court when he considered he was not really needed. This consultant thought that the reason his instructions were often so vague and ill conceived was that he was contracted to provide this service to the local authority; thus, it was considered free at the point of delivery. In effect, the 'issues' in cases were simply presented to him to untangle. This consultant

---

[7] In practice, these fees were met by (what was) the Legal Aid Board, with the solicitor instructed by the guardian undertaking administrative responsibility for negotiating the fee (this Board has been replaced by the CLS – see note 4, Chapter 6).

[8] In practice, the evidence indicates that letters of instruction are generally drafted by solicitors – albeit in consultation with the guardian.

reported some discussion had been undertaken about moving to a position where the local authority had to pay for his services at the point of delivery (i.e. as category 2 work). It was hoped that such a move would encourage the local authority to be more specific about what was required of him. Other consultants complained about inappropriate questions from some local authorities (e.g. questions addressed to the wrong discipline) and tasks posed that were ill defined, that were almost limitless in terms of boundaries and that stretched the expertise of the psychiatrists beyond what they felt able or willing to do.

Further research is therefore necessary to determine whether the quality of instructions tends to be poorer where local health services are contracted to supply a local authority with assessments in the context of legal proceedings.[9] Also, it would be important to ascertain the division of labour between legal services and social services departments in the construction of instructions to experts. In certain authorities, the indications are that this task is increasingly perceived – by legal services departments at least – as the responsibility of lawyers, but there is no national data on practices in this field and anecdotal evidence indicates this may be an area of tension.

Most consultants had undertaken instructions on behalf of parents at some point in their careers, and over half also raised problems in this context. Five consultants were not happy to undertake instructions on behalf of parents because they felt they would not be seen as sufficiently independent and child focused by the court. One national expert said his practice was to "tell parents to go via the court, because I prefer to be seen as child focused". Another consultant said he had now reached a point in his career where he could choose, and he chose not to accept instructions on behalf of parents. A further consultant was critical of the solicitors commonly instructed by parents; he argued that they were not experienced in Children Act proceedings.[10]

Overall, half the consultants said letters of instruction now posed specific questions and this represented some improvement compared with instructions received one or two years previously. However, just

---

[9] And this is particularly the case given subsequent changes as a result of, for example, the new version of *Working Together* (Department of Health *et al*, 2000*b*).
[10] This view concurs with earlier research (see Bates & Brophy, 1996; Brophy & Bates, 1998). However, there were some notable exceptions – and this probably applies in most geographical locations – where the names of certain people and firms of solicitors recur in this type of discussion. For example, one consultant said there were one or two solicitors who worked in an inner-city location with high rates of economic and social deprivation who, despite not being on the Children Panel of the Law Society, were nevertheless experienced as excellent practitioners.

under a third reported that some letters continued to be vague and, as outlined above, this was particularly the case with regard to instructions from certain local authorities – although one consultant said she also considered it part of her job to help the local authority define what it was they wanted from her. Indications were that a minority of psychiatrists continue to receive vague instructions; they may not conform to practices preceding the Children Act (e.g. in effect simply saying 'here are the papers, tell us what you think'), but they may still on occasion request what amounts to the same thing (e.g. 'please give us a psychiatric opinion of this family').

A few consultants had experienced what they called 'being appointed by the court'. One consultant described how a judge had instructed the parties to instruct him in particular in a case:

> "Yes, the judge had got so fed up with the quality of evidence that he'd heard so far, that he decided he wanted somebody who he thought could do the job properly. So, I think every High Court Judge has a list in his head of people who he thinks are competent professional witnesses in child care cases." (N12)

This approach by certain judges was perceived as a considerable compliment by some consultants, but other consultants found that experience somewhat worrying – a reputation as the 'judge's choice' was not necessarily seen as a good thing for a child psychiatrist, because it could compromise views of the procedure and the expert as completely independent.

## *Joint letters of instruction – time for clinicians to debate?*

Most consultants had some experience of receiving a 'joint instruction' on behalf of two or more parties, but, at the time of the interviews at least, this was by no means the most common form of instruction. Moreover, consultants' understandings of what a joint instruction meant and the implications of that approach for both the expert and the parties involved were sometimes vague. Some consultants talked about being the 'agreed' expert, saying this meant all three parties agreed to them as the named expert. But they were less clear about what that indicated in terms of the construction of the questions they were asked to address. Some were not clear about whether all the questions had been mutually agreed or whether parties had added their own questions to a letter from one party only, or whether it simply meant no other party had raised an objection to them as the named choice. For a few consultants, 'joint instructions' and 'agreed instructions' were, in practice, synonymous.[11]

On the whole, at the time of these interviews the national experts gave a clearer view about joint instructions. For them it meant that all parties were clear about why the expert was involved and what the expert was being asked to do. There was, however, less clarity about the implications of that approach with regard to, for example, whether a second opinion would subsequently be possible,[12] and whether it would be necessary for the expert to liaise and record discussions with all advocates (i.e. those other than the 'lead' solicitor), to talk about the outcome with parties, and to take responsibility for discussing the outcome with the parents themselves.

Most consultants saw some of the popular appeal associated with the idea of joint instructions: it indicated a conciliatory approach, at least to the choice of expert; it was seen as better to try to agree on these things; and it was important to try to ensure children were not subjected to multiple assessments. However, in discussing the impact of joint instructions on their profession, some important concerns were raised. Consultants talked about the dangers underlying the appeal of joint instructions and of moving to a culture in which child psychiatrists were prepared to undertake instructions only where they were the agreed expert or where instructions were joint. For example, it indicated their opinions were less likely to be peer reviewed, and interestingly these clinicians saw scrutiny of their work by their peers as a much more demanding, more useful and indeed a more necessary exercise than cross-examination by clever (but nevertheless) lay counsel.

This issue has not received much attention in the UK (cf. Roberts, 1994) but in other jurisdictions it has become the subject of some debate. For example, child neurologists in North American have expressed concerns about the ethics of having a single expert in cases. In a survey of the profession (Child Neurology Society, Ethics and Practice Committee, 1998) two-thirds of clinicians reported that there should be a mechanism for peer review of work and over 50% said

---

[11] During the mid-1990s there was clearly some confusion here. In a national survey of cases, some experts instructed by a guardian were reported as 'agreed' experts but there was no indication that the instructions were 'joint'. Nor, in the majority of these cases (85%), had the court attempted to encourage parties to enter into joint instructions (see Brophy *et al*, 1999*b*, p. 33).

[12] There was, for example, a limited view among consultants that a joint instruction could be a bit like a lottery in which all parties were bound by the outcome and recommendations and would be unable to seek a second opinion. There was also some evidence of that interpretation of the consequences of a joint instruction by a few guardians (Brophy & Bates, 1999).

there should be some monitoring of this work by the Child Neurology Society. While the response rate to the questionnaire was poor (about 25% or 285/1126 members contacted), views demonstrated, from a clinical perspective, the importance of peer review in complex cases, concern regarding the precise role of clinicians in single instructions and a recommendation for reform, with the profession body taking a lead and monitoring this area.

Consultants in this study argued that underlying the immediate appeal of joint instructions there were some possible dangers. A joint instruction *may* meet the needs of policy makers for less costly and possibly quicker proceedings;[13] it may also appear to meet the needs of some overstretched consultants, who sometimes appeared less than enthusiastic about, for example, the prospect of a pre-trial meeting in those (minority of) cases where experts disagree *and* this results in a fully contested final hearing. However, some consultants thought that, as a general practice, joint instructions may herald a loss of 'the critical factor' in proceedings. It may also encourage a view among experts of themselves as being somewhat 'over-precious' in terms of their time and their willingness to submit their work to critical appraisal.

The concerns of consultants about the potential loss of the critical factor in proceedings is underscored by other research where comparisons between potentially competing reports were undertaken based on cases completed by the end of 1994. Tables 8 and 9 demonstrate that disagreement between experts occurs. Indeed, when disagreements and partial disagreements are combined, there was more disagreement than there was full agreement. Moreover, disagreements did not simply occur between experts appointed by the local authority and those appointed by parents: areas of disagreement requiring review and discussion also occurred in cases where the guardian sought a second opinion.

Tables 8 and 9 arguably highlight some of the potential advantages of peer review in complex cases – it also demonstrates that child welfare knowledge is not a unitary category of knowledge. Nevertheless, since the completion of this and other research highlighted above, a number of moves in the Family Division – the most recent being a Practice Direction from the President[14] – have served to increase pressures on

---

[13] Although there are no published comparative data on costs or duration of cases involving the joint instruction of a single expert, the available evidence indicates that, despite the use of joint letters of instruction to one expert, overall, cases continue to increase in duration (Butler-Sloss, 2000).

[14] Practice direction, 25 May 2000, Dame Elizabeth Butler-Sloss, President of the Family Division, *Family Law*, July 2000, p. 509: "... (4) Single Joint Expert (4.1) ... Accordingly where expert evidence is sought to be relied on, parties should

TABLE 8
*The recommendations of experts commissioned by a local authority compared with those commissioned by parents (n = 170)[1]*

|  | Yes (%) | In part (%) | No (%) | NC (%) | NR (%) |
|---|---|---|---|---|---|
| Did 2nd report support any recommendations made by 1st expert? | 41 | 30 | 18 | 6 | 4 |

NC, reports not in practice comparable; NR, no recommendations given in the first report.
1. Sample size was based on those cases where more than one party filed expert evidence and where the guardians identified that the local authority and the parents filed reports that addressed the same issues/concerns.
Source: Brophy *et al* (1999*b*, p. 39).

TABLE 9
*The assessments and recommendations of experts commissioned by a guardian compared with a previous report (n = 78)[1]*

| Comparing | Yes (%) | No (%) | In part (%) | NR (%) |
|---|---|---|---|---|
| *Recommendations* Did recommendations made by guardian's expert (a 2nd opinion) confirm those made in a previous expert's report? (*n* = 68) | 23 | 32 | 19 | 26 |
| *Assessment* Did guardian's expert (a 2nd opinion) support the assessment made in a previous expert's report? (*n* = 74) | 40 | 34 | 26 | N/A |
| *Order* Did guardian's expert support the order requested? (*n* = 67) | 59 | 25 | 16 | N/A |

NR, no recommendations given in the first report.
1. Sample sizes based on 78 cases (after allowing for missing data) where more than one party filed expert reports and where the guardian commissioned further expert evidence on an issue/concern already addressed in an existing report in the case.
Source: Brophy *et al* (1999*b*, p. 40).

if possible agree upon a single expert whom they can jointly instruct. Where parties are unable to agree upon the expert to be instructed, the court will consider using its powers under Part 35 of the Civil Procedure Rules 1998 (SI 1998/3132) to direct that evidence be given by one expert only. In such cases, parties must be in a position at the first appointment or when the matter comes to be considered ... to provide the court with a list of suitable experts or to make submissions as to the method by which the expert is to be selected."

parties to agree jointly to instruct a single expert. Whether and how this practice meets the concerns of these consultants in wishing to retain a critical factor in the work of experts remains questionable and requires further research, particularly perhaps in the light of Article 6 of the Human Rights Act 1998.[15]

But joint instructions may also make it is rather less likely that an expert will be subject to tough cross-examination in the witness box. This is in part because one of the important functions of clinicians giving a second opinion in highly complex cases (e.g. non-accidental injury) is to help the instructing advocate appraise an existing report and construct pertinent questions to be put to its author before a hearing and, if that fails to bring about a negotiated agreement, during cross-examination after giving evidence-in-chief. Some consultants in this study acknowledged that cross-examination in court was probably the least attractive part of their role. Nevertheless, it was perceived as a necessary part of the exercise of trying to get it right for a child and not one easily replaced (see Chapter 5).

## Writing reports for courts

Most consultants interviewed had not received any formal training in writing reports for courts, although most had considerable experience of doing this, both before and after implementation of the Children Act 1989. Most experts saw the main audience for their report as the judge/court. In practice, this meant that attempts were made to write for a non-medical audience, using clear, self-explanatory language and terminology. A few experts also pitched their reports at parents. For example:

> "I tend to frame them as if I were talking primarily to the parents ... I try to make them understand it and try to explore in my report ways in which the family could be helped by reading my report or by the suggestions made for further work." (L14)

But while attempts were made to resist using medical jargon in reports in an effort to make them more accessible to judges, jargon was on occasion used to mask or make more palatable certain issues where parents were concerned:

> "I have nasty little phrases like 'as Mrs "Smith" would be the first to acknowledge etc.' and then I blast her. And sometimes I have to say

---

[15] Article 6 addresses the right of litigants to a fair trial.

> if it's a fairly simple family and I have very unkind things to say, I sometimes jack up the language so that they don't really know what I'm talking about – I write it over their heads." (L6)

This approach may have been adopted by a minority in this sample[16] but it does raise problems if the expert is also expected by an instructing party to go through a report with parents – or to meet with all parties to discuss the report. It may also raise problems for other professionals who undertake this task with parents. Although there does not appear to be any formal guidance on this issue, historically the task has usually fallen to the solicitor representing parents. Experts in this sample were divided as to whether they now saw it as their responsibility to discuss their report and recommendations with parents. For those who felt it was their responsibility, in practice, they described a very ad hoc process of reporting back to parents: it could be by way of a verbal summary at the end of the last session with parents or on the telephone if parents were unhappy with the content of the report, or if parents specifically requested a discussion this could take place in a corridor outside the courtroom. Most of the national experts who saw it as their responsibility to discuss their report with the family qualified this in a number of ways (e.g. when acting on instructions from the local authority, or when specifically requested to discuss the report with parents). When local experts were acting on instructions from a local authority, it was often seen as the responsibility of that authority (the social worker or the solicitor) – or indeed the guardian – to go over the report with parents.

Some consultants were very candid about their feelings about talking to parents – some of whom were likely to be very hostile. This was not seen as a pleasant task and, as with most people, there was a tendency among consultants to want to avoid these confrontations if at all possible. However, it is arguably the case that these specialists may be better at this task, or could be better skilled and trained to undertake it, than other professionals in proceedings (e.g. criminal solicitors acting for parents). This lack of a formal channel for feedback to some parents may mean they do not have sufficient opportunity for discussion and reflection on what they might have to achieve, in terms of their own behaviours, in order to change the recommendations of the expert. Equally, unless they or the professionals request it, parents may not have an opportunity to discuss with a clinician those aspects of the report with which they do not agree or which they feel misrepresent

---

[16] While this particular approach to dealing with 'difficult' parents was not mentioned by other consultants, it cannot be concluded that others may not, on occasion, adopt a similar strategy.

them. Moreover, it may mean certain parents will go on to 'contest the uncontestable'.

Therefore, ensuring formal feedback to parents – arguably by the author of the report but perhaps with some flexibility[17] – appears critical. It could be argued on cost grounds, since it may achieve an uncontested order, but it may also contribute to parents' continued participation in the process of attempting to achieve, if not an agreed outcome, at least one that is better understood. A more formal approach to feedback to parents may also have a potential to improve parents' participation in future care plans for children. In other words, within the principle of partnership with parents wherever possible, it may make some parents at least continue to feel part of the process even when the initial (interim) results seem unlikely to be in their favour.

## *The content of reports and the language of recommendations*

With regard to the content of psychiatric reports for courts, a move towards greater specificity in letters of instruction, coupled with research and training for clinicians in an attempt to encourage the profession 'to get its act together' (e.g. Tufnell, 1993*a*; Tufnell *et al*, 1993, 1996), means that these documents may be in a period of transition. The new legal agenda for Children Act cases, coupled with criticisms of expert reports that conformed to a 'stream of consciousness' approach, has resulted in pressures on clinicians to develop a more focused and analytical style in writing reports. In some cases, as the instructions received by these experts indicated, this can also mean adopting a more legally orientated document. In some instances the experts were being asked, in effect, to move from an arguably strictly clinical arena and a discourse about children's needs and parenting capacities to the legal arena and the technical framework through which those needs might best be met. Thus, some, not surprisingly, were asked to comment on contact issues and on the prospects for future reunification of children with their birth parent(s). Moreover, a majority saw it as part of their task to comment on these issues if they thought it appropriate – whether or not they were requested to do so.

The majority of consultants interviewed would give a view in their report as to whether they thought a court order was necessary, but, as

---

[17] For example, letters of instruction could specify this issue so that all parties were clear regarding who will make an appointment with parents to discuss the report.

reported above, some were more cautious about making a specific recommendation in their report for the court. Most consultants acknowledged having a view of what they thought appropriate in a case, but were nevertheless reluctant to be seen to be "telling a judge what to do" or "stepping on the judge's toes". They might frequently express a view, but most were quick to qualify this with comments such as 'but of course, it is ultimately up to the court to make this decision'. However, as indicated above, judges have on occasion asked experts to express a view on the type of order they think the court should make, and indications are that few child psychiatrists would resist or sit on the fence at that point – most would air their view.

## Using research in court reports – 'evidence-based practice' and strategic planning

The use and applicability of research, at least in reports for courts, remains a contentious issue. Academics in this field have argued some decisions have indicated a failure on the part of courts to take account of relevant research (e.g. Richards, 1988), or that where research has been available to the court, it has been ignored or dismissed (e.g. Golombok & Tasker, 1991; Brophy, 1992).

During the period of this study, two cases in the Family Division addressed the issue of research in expert evidence and it might well be argued that they offer somewhat confusing guidance. In 1991, Mr Justice Cazelet stated, among other things, that experts should:

(a) provide a straightforward, not misleading opinion;
(b) be objective and not omit factors that do not support their opinion;
(c) be properly researched (indicating areas of insufficient data).[18]

The implication here is that relevant research which raises doubts about as well as that which supports the expert's opinion should be included and the expert also has a duty to identify for the court areas where there is insufficient research. The head note for a later case, in 1995, however, might be read as casting some doubt on the use of research. In this case, Mrs Justice Bracewell argued:

"Published material of international research, such as has been produced in this case, is not always helpful to the court, since as Dr

---

[18] *Re R (A Minor) (Expert's Evidence)* [1991] 1 FLR 291.

... pointed out in this case, it is highly selective, often produced to support a particular stance, sometimes on a limited number of specialised cases and further, the conclusions reached may depend on a diagnosis which involves assumptions about the underlying history which gave rise to the injury in each of the cases studied and which may not have been tested evidentially or established in fact. I did not, for those reasons, derive much assistance in this case from the research produced."[19]

Arguably, Mrs Justice Bracewell's comments here refer to the selective and inappropriate use of research, and not to the use of research *per se*. The fact that the judge later stated that she was in fact "impressed with the practical research" undertaken by one expert witness[20] adds weight to this interpretation. The Children Act Advisory Committee's (1997) best practice guidance supports this interpretation. Drawing on the views of Mr Justice Cazelet, it states that where expert opinion is based, wholly or in part, on research conducted by others, the expert must state this in the report and identify the research.[21] Thus, research continues to have a relevance – albeit only if it seems that an "expert opinion is based, wholly or in part, on it".

Experts in this study were divided as to the use of research in their reports. But their responses owed more to the development of strategies for dealing with lawyers in court and time constraints on their work[22] than to guidance from case law. Overall, just over half the sample indicated that they did refer to relevant research in their reports. These consultants considered it part of their job and part of their 'added value', hence they considered it their responsibility to know the relevant research and to be able to discuss it and demonstrate its particular relevance to the court.

The remainder of the sample, however, either seldom referred to research or used it only when they considered it was unavoidable. Some consultants said research very much informed their work, although they might not explicitly mention this in reports – it was more likely to come up in discussions. Others were more anxious about the use and

---

[19] *Manchester City Council* v. *B* [1995] 1 FLR 324 – head note.

[20] In a case of alleged non-accidental injury this expert, a paediatric radiologist, was reported as having undertaken some research focusing on the relationship between minor damage and subdural haematomas, and the sample size was reported as some 2300 (*Manchester City Council* v. *B* [1995] 1 FLR 329f). It is not, however, clear from the reported case whether this research had been published and thus subject to the normal channels of scientific review.

[21] CAAC (1997:28) *Handbook of Best Practice in Children Act Cases,* London: Lord Chancellor's Department.

[22] One consultant thought its omission was probably due to a degree of laziness.

misuse of research in the legal arena. Finding research that was relevant, taking research out of context and the dangers of being upstaged by "some smart lawyer who is always able to find research that says something else" were posed as reasons for not including research. In effect, using research in reports could be a risky strategy, as one consultant argued:

> "you're playing the game with the lawyers if you start throwing papers around." (L10)

Ad hoc evidence indicates that other experts have questioned whether it is their job to identify and comment on findings from research other than their own. That particular approach raises some worrying questions about 'evidence-based practice' in the child protection arena and the development of approaches that attempt to integrate individual clinical practice and what has been called 'the best external evidence' (e.g. Sackett *et al*, 1996). It also begs a question: if it is not the job of the child psychiatrist who offers expertise as an expert witness for the court to be up to date on relevant research and to be able to draw on that body of knowledge and to point out its relevance for the court, it is difficult to see just whose task that should be. The consultants interviewed in this study considered research skills and knowledge to be part of their 'added value' to proceedings and, thus, it was their responsibility to be up to date on the relevant research. They differed, however, as to whether that information should be included in the report itself.[23]

## 'On the receiving end': improvements to the work of experts following the 1989 Children Act

As outlined in Table 5 (Chapter 2), the majority of consultants in this study had had experience as an expert witness both before and after implementation of the Children Act, and consultants were able to

---

[23] It is also the case that other professionals, for example certain social workers, guardians, psychologists and academic researchers, have argued that they are at least as well equipped as a child psychiatrist to comment on relevant research. The issue remains debatable as members of each profession claim some expertise in this field. However, in the context of the overall package that these specialists are being asked to provide, and in view of their responsibility to the court, it is arguably appropriate that they should comment on the research evidence informing their opinions and on the evidence that might undermine their views. That approach lies at the heart of evidence-based practice in this field.

---

Box 3
*Improvements to care proceedings after the Children Act 1989:
views and experiences of child psychiatrists*

- Increased dialogue with experts.
- Pre-trial meetings between experts who disagree.
- Improved letters of instruction.
- Improvements in the reports written by experts.
- The development of a more critical perspective by experts to their own work.
- Improvements to practices resulting from the use of specialist solicitors from the Children Panel of the Law Society.
- Some improvements in working with parents.

---

identify a number of improvements when comparing practices in the two periods (Box 3).

One of the major achievements of the Children Act has been to increase the dialogue with experts. This change was viewed as one of the most substantial achievements and improvements were identified on several levels: between experts themselves, between experts and instructing parties, and between experts and the court.[24] Where consultants had been involved in cases in which conflicting evidence had been filed, they reported that meetings between experts had, on the whole, identified and reduced areas of conflict. What could not be ascertained from this type of study, however, and what is important given the findings in Tables 8 and 9, was the consequences of those negotiations – for the children and parents concerned and for the order finally made by the court.

Although, as identified above, there remained room for improvement in letters of instruction from some local authorities and advocates for parents, on the whole consultants reported that letters of instruction were continuing to improve. Not surprisingly, these child psychiatrists also argued that, where instruction had improved, their court reports had also improved.

Experts also reported that they were now forced to think about issues in more depth and to question their own opinions and the evidence on which those opinions were based. Like guardians (see Brophy & Bates, 1998), experts also felt that specialist solicitors could make an enormous contribution to improving the quality of the work of the expert witness. Moreover, in those instances where local authorities

---

[24] Although it should be noted the study identified room for improvement in dialogue with parents, given some experts' reluctance to accept instructions on behalf of parents or to discuss their reports with them.

had been more willing to consider changing their choice of expert, for example where that choice was unacceptable to parents, experts considered that flexibility had made a contribution to improving things. There is, however, only limited evidence of this shift of stance by some local authorities. This is a complex issue, which requires further research.

In summary, despite the fact that many of the changes to the role and responsibilities of experts did not take into account the structures or contractual obligations of many clinicians, or the difficulties that many CAMHS were undergoing in terms of the loss of resources and staff, on the whole many of the changes following the Children Act were welcomed and, in the opinion of these consultants at least, have improved many aspects of their work for courts in cases of child abuse, neglect or maltreatment.

# 5 A new clinical agenda: challenges for child protection litigation

## Introduction

As outlined in Chapter 1, taken together, the principles that under-scored the Children Act 1989 and the subsequent directions for good practice in cases involving experts indicate that 'law' is carving out a new agenda for clinicians instructed as expert witnesses. However, in exploring the issues that have driven this change, it is important to understand that some child welfare specialists have been centrally involved in parts of that process. This applies both in relation to substantive developments in case law and in the wider child protection arena,[1] but also with regard to the forum in which policy issues are debated and developed.[2]

In other words, the relationship between 'law' and child welfare knowledge is now multi-layered and cannot be viewed as one in which 'law' will inevitably dominate child welfare knowledge. Research and policy following the Children Act confirm that the contemporary family justice system is without doubt a multi-disciplinary enterprise.

---

[1] That is, as this chapter demonstrates, experts serve an educational function within individual cases in which they are instructed, but their influence is also *possible* in the early stages in the child protection investigation process, for example on local authority area child protection committees.

[2] For example, the President's Interdisciplinary Family Law Committee, and its Education and Training Sub-Committee, but also in para-legal form, for example those commissioned by central government departments to develop and write part of the new *Framework for the Assessment of Children in Need and Their Families* (Department of Health *et al*, 2000*a*) and supporting questionnaires and scales (Department of Health *et al*, 2000*c*) *The Family Assessment Pack of Questionnaires and Scales*. Also, of course, doctors are employed as senior policy advisers within the NHS Executive.

This is not to suggest, however, that the relationship (both within and outside the courts) is without tensions or conflict – or that limited resources do not ultimately determine policy agenda in both camps. The justifications for and pressures upon parties to agree to a joint letter of instruction to a single expert, and the continued exclusion of public law work from much mainstream NHS work despite the promise of further funding of some £84 million for CAMHS made in the spring of 2000 (see Chapter 6) might arguably demonstrate the supremacy of the cost factor over both discourses. However, the interface of the two discourses occurs at a number of levels in modern government and indications are that the outcome – at least in terms of any clash of discourses – is much less predictable than previous writers have suggested.

This chapter explores experts' views about their own work in the legal arena. While 'law' continues to carve out a new agenda for experts, the views and experiences of these consultants demonstrate that child psychiatrists are also developing something of an agenda for their work in child protection litigation. Moreover, this agenda may not conform with what advocates or indeed courts consider most appropriate.

First, the tensions between a forensic and a therapeutic orientation to this work are explored. Second, the issue of competing expert opinion is addressed along with views about both why these occur and whether they usually represent common disputes between established, known camps in this field. Views about new procedures for addressing differences – for example, the instigation of meetings of experts before the final trial – are also explored. Third, consultants addressed the complex issue (at least for lawyers) of notions of 'hard' and 'soft' evidence in this field and views that their work has traditionally been regarded as falling into the latter category. And, in the light of much discussion and some misunderstanding about inquisitorial and adversarial proceedings, interviews explored with consultants their views and experiences of cross-examination in court. Finally, in weighing up the impact of the Children Act 1989, consultants outlined their criticisms and areas of disappointment with proceedings under the Act. As these consultants demonstrate, there is much in this emerging clinical agenda that requires wider debate.

## The 'forensic' exercise and children's future therapeutic needs: a need for debate

As indicated in Chapter 3, instructions from parties usually asked child psychiatrists to address children's future therapeutic needs. Where they did not, consultants would usually comment on this issue and most included recommendations about future therapeutic work in their report for the court. Two issues arose in discussions about the future therapeutic needs of children following physical or sexual abuse or neglect or maltreatment by their parents. The first issue related to the basis on which recommendations for treatment should be made. The second was concerned with determining the relationship between the forensic exercise and any future therapeutic input.

The question of whether recommendations for future treatment of children were based solely on an assessment of clinical need, or whether they were based on the resources known to be available locally, revealed a problematic area for consultants. The national experts were divided: half made recommendations solely on the basis of assessed need and half made recommendations based on both need and likely available local resources. This apparent divergence of approach, however, was not because some national experts were unaware of what a local CAMHS could provide (i.e. geographical location did not influence the recommendations). Rather, it was influenced by matters of clinical need and a desire therefore to set out in principle the services and support a child and possibly carers required. Two of the national experts thought it important to record both categories of information in reports, identifying what was necessary and what was likely to happen in a case. This approach was deemed important on two grounds: first, with regard to what was most likely to happen with regard to meeting children's therapeutic needs following maltreatment by parents or carers; and second, because of the likely impact on the locally based consultant/services. As one consultant argued:

> "I will never go to a place and recommend something which I haven't checked out first as being available [because] it drives me crazy when I can't do a job here because I'm too busy, so the local authority gets somebody in from miles away, that person [makes] a whole set of recommendations about a family which nobody can provide. What use is that to a court?" (N12)

Most local experts expressed anxieties about trying to pitch recommendations somewhere between a clinical assessment of need and knowledge of limited local resource, but also about making recommendations that another clinician would be expected to take forward. For example:

> "Yes, I do make recommendation [on treatment]. It's horrible. I often get asked to make recommendations and I'll ring the shrink in the area and say this is the problem etc. and then I trail my coat into the court ... I will be asked to write a letter of referral, because

if I don't write it, they [the local authority] won't do it – I know
from experience. Of course, we clinicians hate having work imposed
on us by some distant person in a court: you think, stuff that, but if
you've agreed to it beforehand, then. ... " (L6)

This consultant was not alone in expressing frustration at the paucity
of resources for therapeutic services for children, compared, for
example, with the cost of legal proceedings. For example:

"I remember being in court and the recommendation I made for a
child was going to cost £3000 and the local authority said they didn't
have the money, so I said, 'Well, I will forego my court fee in this
case if anybody else in the room would be prepared to do the same'.
There was a lot of uncomfortable shuffling and a few phone calls,
and then the local authority decided they could afford it. The
absurd thing is that the whole case had cost far more than the
therapy would have cost. ... "

This clinician, however, was unable to offer much herself in the way
of follow-up treatment for the children she assessed within court
proceedings. She continued:

"We are badly served locally. We don't have an adolescent unit. We
have to post all our in-patient kids over the borders... We have one
child guidance clinic ... but the fact that we have a good child
guidance clinic here highlights how bad everything else is because
if we don't do it, nothing gets done."[3] (L6)

In practice, most of the local experts ended up making recommendations for follow-up treatment that were a combination of assessed
clinical need and what they knew to be available in local services. Only
two local experts said they would make recommendations solely on
the basis of need, leaving it to the local authority to locate the necessary
resources and services.

A second set of concerns arising out of discussions about the future
therapeutic needs for children centred on the relationship between
certain types of forensic work and any future treatment. As identified
above, there was some concern about the professional ethics of a
consultant making recommendations that another clinician would
have to take up. One consultant in this sample said she would not
make any recommendations about follow-up treatment for this

---

[3] This consultant was due to retire shortly after the interview and expressed grave
concern about what would happen to the limited service in that geographical area
once that happened.

reason. Others argued that the forensic exercise should be separate from any future treatment, and the same consultant should not undertake both tasks. For example:

> "I take referrals on to write reports ... there was one where there was an implicit request that I would take them [the children] on after I'd done the report. I made it clear to everyone that I was writing the report but if I decided the children needed therapeutic input – it wouldn't be undertaken by me." (L7)

Other consultants, however, had begun to question the ethics of separating these tasks. They thought it was potentially damaging, and thus unethical for them as doctors, to make recommendations for children without offering any treatment. Some consultants said ideally they would prefer to see referrals in child protection litigation in terms of a potential package, indicating, if necessary, an ongoing commitment to treat a child:

> "I find it quite damaging, the idea of having these cases then not sometimes continuing to work with them. I'd prefer to have a small group of cases ... and [be able to take] the child and the necessary work forward." (N16)

> "It's one of the reasons that I mostly do local work because I feel strongly that if one is going to get embroiled with people for assessments ... for courts, then one ought to be prepared to follow through and you can't do that if people live at the other end of the country." (L9)

A number of factors influenced whether these consultants could in practice offer any future therapeutic input. First, if consultants were doing the court work privately (e.g. if they had retired from NHS practice or were academics without a clinical case-load) they were unable to offer any follow-up work. Second, although a majority of the consultants based in local services thought they would be able to offer *some* further follow-up work, or said they would try hard to stick with the children, in practice, in hard-pressed services, this work had a lower clinical priority than other work.[4] As consultants indicated above, the kind of follow-up work that was likely to be needed after care

---

[4] This is an issue that requires further research. Little is known about follow-up work with these children. Available research suggests that good intentions are unlikely to be enough. For example, in a national survey of guardians the majority (72%) reported that one of the major problems they experienced with local CAMHS was a lack of resources or commitment to undertake further therapeutic work if that was deemed necessary (Brophy *et al*, 1999*b*, p. 12).

proceedings was often not centrally concerned with mental health issues as such. Thus, in a resource-starved service, children with more immediate, life-threatening mental health problems would generally take clinical priority.

### Working for the court or working for the child?

When instructed in care proceedings, consultants considered they were working for the court, but, as clinicians, they also considered they had an independent duty of care to the child. Before the final hearing (e.g. in discussing instructions, assessments, writing the report for the court, pre-hearing meetings), these child welfare specialists did not indicate that their approach or their child welfare knowledge, their discourse, became subordinated or subservient to a legal discourse. They did not indicate that current pre-hearing practices, in effect, reduced their work to 'cogs in the wheel' of a (dominating) legal process as they struggled to meet a different conceptual framework that law is said to impose on clinicians. Indeed, they may not have set the legal wheel in motion but, once involved, discussions indicated that confidence in their status, expertise and knowledge, coupled with a very strong desire to get it right – or as near right as possible for the individual child – meant they had little apprehension, and certainly nothing that could be described as trepidation, in attempting to influence or shift the direction of analysis if they considered parties were on the wrong track.

## Competing expert opinions

Most of the consultants interviewed had some experience of cases in which there was a degree of conflict between the views of appointed experts. In line with contemporary practices, most consultants had also entered into discussions with other experts in order to clarify areas of agreement and disagreement for the court, and to identify those issues that the court would likely have to resolve at the final hearing.[5]

The national experts in this sample were more likely to have undertaken these negotiations by telephone and letter than by meeting in person. This may be a feature of the geographical distances between experts. But geographical location could also be

---

[5] The aim of these meetings being to narrow down disagreements or, more hopefully, by reaching some further agreement to render at least some of the oral evidence unnecessary.

an issue for local consultants. One consultant in particular identified the difficulties and the implications for his general clinical practice of trying to negotiate in person:

> "it's an enormous burden, you can imagine, working in a region as big as this … this is a recommendation that stems out of London, where, if you happen to be at Kings, or Westminster, or Guy's or 'Tommy's', people are around the corner. … I've actually got to cancel a whole day's work and the other expert has to do the same for us to meet somewhere in the middle of [this] region." (L15)

On the whole, consultants thought that, where competing expert evidence was filed, most responsible psychiatrists would do their best to try to narrow down the differences. Sometimes it appeared differences were more apparent than real:

> "people say to you, in private, this woman's a real toe-rag or this father's a crook, or whatever, but when we really sort of, get off our 'high horses' … we may differ in our optimism as to the outcome, but the differences are usually quite small." (L6)

Nevertheless, it was felt important for consultants to address these issues directly:

> "Yes, it's the best bit of work if you can actually thrash out the problems. … But the barristers don't like it because we can actually come up with a consensus, which cuts the cash short, and I wonder whether judges like it." (L3)

These views about the relative magnitude of conflicts – but also about the value of working through differences of opinion – were endorsed by some national experts. They also thought that some of the differences of opinion were quite small, albeit, not surprisingly, these were usually exploited by lawyers.

The objective of meetings between experts is to identify the sources of conflict and areas of agreement, but guardians have suggested that such meetings have a range of additional important benefits, and these are listed in Box 4.

Guardians used these meetings to explore with experts their real knowledge of the child and family (and this was especially the case where guardians considered assessments had been something of a snapshot). But meetings also afforded an opportunity to consider the existence of any vested interests, such as whether one expert was in the pocket of the local authority, or whether the other expert was trying to be nice to the parents. They also enabled guardians to challenge experts where they perceived gaps between the evidence in

---

Box 4
*Pre-trial meetings with experts: benefits and opportunities*

- The testing of 'grounded' knowledge of a child and his or her family.
- The location of any vested interests.
- The exploration of the relationship between evidence and opinion.
- A final 'mediation' opportunity.
- The exploration of whether treatment or services recommended for a family are a real option.
- The testing of whether reports have a research input.

Source: Brophy & Bates (1999).

---

reports and the final opinions expressed, and to identify or clarify the basis of certain opinions expressed. Meetings also offered guardians a last opportunity to ascertain whether issues could be narrowed down, to check what was now non-negotiable and where there might be room for manoeuvre.

Like some of the consultants above, guardians were also concerned to check whether any treatment or support recommendations made by the expert were realistic. Thus, guardians also used these meetings to discover, for example, what treatment and further assessment facilities existed locally. And meetings provided an opportunity to address any issues raised by relevant research and, if necessary, to explore the implications of this research for the case with experts.

However, once in court, clinicians fully accepted that it was the job of advocates to identify and exploit any remaining conflict to the best advantage of their clients and thus arguably to undermine or at least cast some doubt on the opinion and recommendations of an expert in the eyes of the court. And, indeed, most consultants in this study saw that as an *appropriate* task of the advocate: 'that's their job – that's what they're paid for'. In other words, challenge and rigorous cross-examination to test the validity of opinions were expected by these clinicians.

The format of pre-trial meetings attended by these consultants varied. Some meetings were attended by experts only, some were attended by experts and advocates, and some were attended by the guardian. Some selected their own chair and some were chaired by the guardian or the solicitor for the child. In principle, this variation in format may not be a problem: it may not need to be too formal and, indeed, a lack of formality *may* be one of its chief benefits. However, as guardians have argued, such meetings should not become mini-trials.

Where things started to go wrong during a meeting, the lack of an independent chair could, as one consultant argued, prove disastrous.

One consultant in particular argued strongly that these meetings should be chaired by the guardian. This was for two reasons. First, it was argued that guardians were the only party with a complete overview of the case – they have access to all documentation, have seen all the local authority files and have talked to all the relevant parties. Second, the guardian was considered independent. This consultant had experienced lawyers attempting to stop a guardian attending meetings of experts, arguing that it was the lawyers' job.[6]

### 'Do you come here often?' Competing paradigms and the known adversary

There is some evidence in both case law and research (Brophy & Bates, 1998) that certain experts have become identified with certain parties and with particular views. Consultants were therefore asked whether they thought they were known for particular views and whether, when issues were contested, they frequently came up against the same colleagues in court. More national than local experts said they frequently came up against the same expert in proceedings. Only a few local experts identified experts whom they tended to come up against more often than others. But, as one consultant in this latter group said, in practice this experience may be more closely associated with the small number of consultants in the 'patch' than with the ideas and views with which each may be associated.

Two features arose in discussions with national experts about their experiences of cases where conflicting opinions were filed. First, their wider, national experience meant that they were more familiar with some of the figures on the national network. Second, they were also aware of the research and clinical interests of people on this network.

Other writers in the field of expert witnesses and child abuse have argued that it is a natural human trait to view as unbiased that opinion with which one agrees and to see others as biased or lacking independence (e.g. Keenan & Williams, 1993).[7] In the field of child

---

[6] There was some guidance with regard to these meetings at the time of the interviews. For example, in *Re C (Expert Evidence: Disclosure Practice)* [1995] 1 FLR 204, it was stated that it should be a condition of appointment of any experts that they should be required to hold discussions with other experts, and that there should be a coordinator for these meetings, such as the guardian ad litem. Subsequently, more formal parameters have been set for the conduct of these meetings, with a suggestion that they are most productive when chaired by a lawyer (Wall, 2000).

[7] Although it might well be argued here that one of the central issues is one of understanding and demonstrating scientific method in the work that underscores opinions.

abuse, although professional protocol (and fear of libel suits) makes some expert witnesses more cautious than others in discussing these issues, there was some very frank discussion of developments in this area and what was termed the 'rent a doc division'. These latter consultants were seen by some of the interviewees as being on a campaign. For example, it was argued that certain experts think parents or fathers in particular get a bad deal in court, or they are known constantly to disagree with paediatric opinion about whether an injury was likely to have been non-accidental, or routinely to recommend trying rehabilitation of children and parents, or to encourage parents to 'contest the uncontestable'. There were a few experts whom interviewees continued to meet during care proceedings who still had difficulty believing that child sexual abuse actually happens. As one consultant in this sample argued when discussing the possibility of meeting a known adversary in legal proceedings:

> "The truly independent experts don't have any difficulty ... The difficulty is when you encounter these people who one might call 'rent a doc'; for example, there is an infamous doctor who will invariably argue. ... " (N12)

Asked whether they themselves might be identified with any particular views, consultants were remarkably frank – most of the national experts thought they were probably identified with certain views. Discussions covered a wide range of issues about contact with children in care, about the viability of rehabilitation of children with parents following abuse (e.g. where there had been no acknowledgement of responsibility or at least culpability), and about issues surrounding fostering and open adoption.

Fewer than half the local experts thought they were also probably identified with particular views, although some thought they might be viewed as overly optimistic in their recommendations and others as very pessimistic. For example:

> "Oh, I think I'm probably seen as quite tough, you know, taking kids away a lot I imagine." (L10)

Some consultants linked the issue of whether they were known for particular views within the child protection arena with the reputation likely to have been acquired as a result of the parties from whom they generally accepted instructions. For example, routinely accepting instructions from the local authority only may result in a reputation for, at best, usually supporting the local authority's application or, at worst, being in the pocket of the local authority.

However, what most consultants also tried to emphasise was their attempt to be balanced as much as their willingness to fight for parents, or to have an openness with regard to rehabilitation or contact, and that this did not necessarily indicate predictability:

> "There are times when I feel I am the person who fights very hard against the local authority on behalf of the parents, and other times when I think I'm the one who takes their kids away from them – it just depends on the run of cases you get ... but I *hope* I come across as neutral." (L19)

As mentioned above, most of the local experts did not think they were associated with particular views – or hoped they were not. That perception may arise because (compared with the national group) this group of consultants undertook fewer cases per year and were unlikely to undertake any research and publishing in this field. Thus, compared with consultants working on a national basis and undertaking many cases per year, it is unlikely that trends could be identified from their work or views hypothesised on the basis of publications or previous reports.

In addition, the heavy emphasis on the need for independence and objectivity from experts in recent years has resulted in a degree of resistance to looking at the construction of neutrality in this field or how reputation is a social construction frequently beyond the immediate control of consultants themselves. Also, the development of certain reputations may be inevitable, given the nature of the issues and the small number of consultants working in this area. One consultant reported being surprised to discover, from a chance conversation, that she was identified with mothers. This was not how she would describe herself. But reputation does not necessarily mean the same thing as predictability (i.e. the degree to which a clinician can be relied upon to give broadly the same opinion about certain issues in most cases).

Nevertheless, there is something of a paradox here. Certainty may be what the legal system or at least the advocate has traditionally sought from the expert witness. Guardians, for example, have identified, as one of their selection criteria, wanting someone who can withstand cross-examination in the witness box – someone who can hold their ground under challenge. Conversely, or perhaps perversely, it may not enhance the consultant's reputation in general where this perceived strength becomes associated with a degree of dogged intransigence or predictability. Equally, if during cross-examination experts are asked a particularly difficult question, where the response is likely to have implications for their opinion and recommendations, experts are now also encouraged to ask a judge for time to think, or even for a short adjournment. In other words, experts clearly have to walk a very fine line in this area and the pressures, not always in the same direction, are considerable. One consultant was particularly frank about the reputation he thought he had acquired regarding certain issues that arise in most care proceedings:

> "Oh, certainly, I mean, I make no bones about it, I'm an accused person ... what I've noticed is ... that you'll be used for a while and then nobody wants you ... but then, after a gap, I'll be approached again." (N18)

## The 'texture' of expert evidence

Despite debates between clinicians themselves about what constitutes 'hard' and 'soft' evidence, 'law', or perhaps more accurately legal method, continues to look for hard evidence and to seek some certainty from psychiatric and psychological experts. In the American literature, one example of the impact of this pressure has been the increased trend to attempt to present mental health evidence in the form of physical forensic evidence. This, it is argued, has the effect of translating the soft evidence of the mental health assessment into hard evidence for the purposes of legal proceedings. Thus, descriptions of the 'battered child syndrome' and the 'sexual abuse accommodation syndrome' aim to provide the court with a 'medicalised' profile of the behaviour of children that is typically consistent with having been physically or sexually abused (e.g. Sagatun, 1991).

Findings from this study, however, indicate that, in this jurisdiction at least (i.e. in England and Wales), the debate on what constitutes hard evidence, and comparisons between certain types of physical medical evidence as hard and mental health evidence as soft may be taking a different path. Instead of attempting to present all evidence as a variation on one arguably problematic model drawn from the physical sciences, child psychiatrists appear to be mounting some resistance to the way in which these issues have been constructed and understood. Within the clinical agenda identified in these interviews, there was a strong emphasis on trying to *educate* courts and lawyers about the particular nature of their field of expertise, the kinds of knowledge they offer and the validation of the conclusions they draw.

This is not to say that in the UK experts do not continue to express exasperation with lawyers who require an oversimplified version of medical evidence (e.g. James, 1995, p. 52). Neither does it imply that the debate over hard and soft evidence does not continue, particularly in the field of child sexual abuse, although, as Roberts argues (1994), "there is little in the field of child sexual abuse which can be said ... with reasonable medical certainty". Rather, these interviews indicate that some child psychiatrists are dealing with it somewhat differently – in effect they are trying to change the parameters of the debate by attacking the dichotomy itself.

First, consultants were asked whether there were pressures on them to oversimplify evidence or to make categorical statements in child protection litigation. Surprisingly, most had not had much recent experience of either of these pressures. There were instances where, under pressure from lawyers, consultants found themselves becoming more dogmatic, or where they felt they were being pushed to a conclusion they did not feel was justified, or where lawyers tried to create or exploit minor differences – what one consultant called "nit picking about small pieces of data … without necessarily debating the larger picture". But while criticisms continue to be made of the use of criminal lawyers in this field, many consultants were impressed with the ability of specialist lawyers to understand the models and theoretical frameworks that underscored their work. For example:

> "I never cease to be amazed at how competent good child care lawyers are in grasping the important basic issues." (L15)

While most consultants were very interested in the question of whether their work constituted 'soft' evidence and the issues it raised in relation to the presentation of their assessments and skills for courts, interestingly, many were entirely comfortable with a description of the kind of evidence they provided as 'soft', if that meant that, in the final analysis, it was interpretive. There were no attempts to present work in what one described as "some pseudo-scientific" framework. They argued that their opinions – for example about whether a parent had the capacity, ability and willingness to change and to do this within a time frame that was meaningful for the child (in terms of his or her developmental needs) – were based on professional judgements rather than something that could be objectively proved. Consultants saw it as part of their task to educate courts about their methods of assessment and the information on which their judgements were based. For example, one consultant talked at length about the diagnosis of emotional abuse and evidence of such maltreatment and how this might differ from evidence produced in cases of, for example, physical abuse, where a photograph of a bruise, or burns, or a radiograph showing new and older healing fractures might suffice. As this consultant acknowledged:

> "You can't take a photograph of a mother shouting at a child." (N18)

But this consultant saw it as part of her job to educate courts both about the assessment exercise necessary to establish whether a child's treatment by a parent amounted to emotional abuse and about the damage and the long-term effects of this type of maltreatment on a child's health and development. This type of maltreatment and its assessment have been controversial, but many consultants felt that the term emotional abuse[8] is now much more acceptable and increasingly better understood by courts than it was a few years previously.

So, for example, in trying to create a framework in which courts could understand the circumstances and needs of the child, most consultants argued that child abuse does not occur in a vacuum. As outlined in Chapter 3, consultants said that it was rare for a child to suffer sexual abuse alone; it is more usual for there to be multiple levels of maltreatment. Thus, a child who suffers physical and/or sexual abuse is also likely to suffer emotional abuse.[9] Some consultants expressed concern about what they felt was a recent overemphasis by courts on 'evidence' in sexual abuse cases. They were concerned that local authorities were not initiating proceedings sufficiently early because of fears that they lacked sufficient evidence to prove sexual abuse. These consultants argued that some of the cases referred to them should have been brought earlier, on the grounds of emotional abuse. One consultant in particular said she preferred to focus on emotional abuse and the quality of parenting in such cases, partly because of the difficulty of meeting the high burden of proof required in sexual abuse cases,[10] and partly because of the need to emphasise the importance of the whole parent/child relationship as the critical factor in sexual abuse cases. The search for a diagnostic label can be useful, but it was also argued by some of these consultants that this exercise could be overvalued.[11]

In other words, presenting their work as interpretive was not, in principle, perceived as a problem, in terms of either validity or mode of presentation. In discussing these issues one consultant was critical of what she described as the 'pseudo-science' of psychometric testing often provided by psychologists. For these child psychiatrists, the task, indeed the challenge, was to unpack and explain their approach and

---

[8] Or 'psychological maltreatment', as some clinicians prefer to call it (e.g. Jones, 1991). A number of clinicians argue that this form of abuse may be at least as important as sexual or physical abuse (e.g. Jones & Alexander, 1987; Bentovim, 1990; Claussen & Crittenden, 1991).

[9] Figures for 1990, published in Hobbs & Wynne (1990), support this view.

[10] See *Re H (Minors) (Sexual Abuse: Standard of Proof)* (1996) 2 WLR 8; and Burrows (1996).

[11] And it could of course be argued that this dilemma illustrates one of the tensions between the discourses of child welfare knowledge and 'law', one focusing on the picture as a whole (the child within his or her world), the other, emanating from 'law', searching for a diagnostic label and evidence as the starting point.

their methods to the court, not to repackage it as something it was not, simply to meet the demands of a debate or criteria with which they did not necessarily agree. One consultant argued that it was because of the very interpretive nature of the evidence that experts produce in this field that the number of experts in cases should not be artificially limited. He argued that in highly complex cases it was in the interests of the child and the court to hear more than one opinion and to make an assessment of the relative merits of the arguments tendered.

Although consultants were critical of aspects of proceedings under the Children Act (see Box 5 below), this was not based on the view that courts did not appear to value, or attempt to understand, interpretive evidence in the context of child and family functioning. Consultants were not being increasingly pressurised to present their evidence in the form of 'hard' evidence, and they appeared on the whole to reject such divisions as not being particularly helpful in the context of the Children Act and the significant harm criteria. Rather, they reported that courts demonstrated increased respect for and understanding of the type of child welfare knowledge they brought. It was their extensive training and range of clinical expertise that added value to their judgements, but also, of course, professional prestige and high social status undeniably lent substantial authority to their judgements. There remains some pressure under heavy cross-examination to move beyond their evidence and area of expertise, but bitter experiences in court (or baptism by fire as it was sometimes called) had taught consultants not only the pitfalls of doing so but also, importantly, how to handle that kind of pressure in future.[12]

**Why test the evidence of experts?**
**The adversarial experience revisited**

One of the objectives of the Children Act 1989 was to continue a trend towards a more inquisitorial style of proceedings in cases concerning children. Previously, it had been argued that it was the very adversarial nature of proceedings that resulted in some specialists refusing to undertake medico-legal work (Lloyd-Bostock, 1988; Carson, 1990; King, 1991). Consultants were therefore asked whether they thought there had been changes, particularly with regard to their experiences in court under cross-examination. As outlined in

---

[12] Training courses and seminars have been developed by both academics and lawyers that specifically focus on coaching experts on how to present their evidence, deal with difficult questions and handle cross-examination where the aim may be to distort or misrepresent their evidence (e.g. 'Developing Witness Skills' – Behavioural Science and Law Network, University of Southampton).

the introduction (p. xix), previous literature (Lloyd-Bostock, 1988; Brophy *et al*, 1999*b*; King, 1991) indicated that courtroom experiences were likely to be an area of concern and continued criticism from clinicians.

In practice, consultants thought care proceedings remained essentially adversarial. However, they were remarkably uncritical of that practice. They identified a number of factors that have mitigated the adversarial nature of final hearings; for example, as outlined above, pre-trial meetings where potentially competing reports have been filed have reduced the number issues to be fought out in court. This has resulted in less room for barristers to nit-pick or cross-examine on minor differences of opinion. Also, consultants thought that the use of specialist advocates[13] reduced unnecessarily aggressive cross-examination. In particular, it was also reported that a good judge would exert control in court where cross-examination became too personalised. However, consultants readily accepted that while children cases were meant to be non-adversarial, this did not mean that witnesses should not be subject to rigorous cross-examination.

These consultants also argued that doctors have always been accorded a great deal of respect and courtesy in court when compared with, for example, social workers, health visitors or nurses. Consultants reported that in their experience these latter groups of professionals were, on the whole, given a much rougher time under cross-examination and were subjected to a far more aggressive style of cross-examination from advocates than would be attempted with doctors.

Some consultants acknowledged that being cross-examined in the witness box remained the least enjoyable aspect of their role in public law work.[14] The majority were, nevertheless, emphatic: their evidence should be challenged in court – indeed, it was essential. For example:

> "I deserve all I get in the witness box; judges know they don't have to look after me." (N12)

Consultants felt that the knowledge that they could be rigorously cross-examined ensured a well-disciplined framework. It provided an important background against which they constructed their reports, and they considered it could be a good test of their knowledge and

---

[13] That is, solicitors on the Children Panel of the Law Society and barristers specialising in family law. It should be noted, however, that while there is a system of accreditation for solicitors wishing to work in this field, there is at present no similar system for barristers.

[14] Although two consultants reported they enjoyed the experience, one said he actually felt outdone if he did not get his day in court, and an opportunity to "strut [his] stuff".

judgements. It could bring out many points. It also forced them to use their skills and expertise to present evidence and opinion from a common-sense angle. It was a challenge to their profession, although not necessarily one that many consultants could, or indeed would, tolerate:

> "I think it's important because I'm so aware of experts who never think, and the one thing that I've learned through forensic work is that all professionals have a great deal to think about. Far too many doctors, particularly specialist doctors, are like little tinpot gods and it's very [pause], a lot of doctors refuse to give evidence because they find it so humiliating." (N18)

Also, as other clinicians have argued (e.g. Wolkind, 1994), it is easy for an individual to develop a rigid and possibly idiosyncratic set of practices and viewpoints, which are applied to all cases. Thus, although giving evidence-in-chief and being cross-examined were not entirely 'enjoyable' experiences, they were nevertheless seen as fundamental to the process. Indeed, some consultants felt that at times they were given too gentle a ride, were treated as too precious and too respectfully, and were sometimes not sufficiently challenged in court:

> "I'm delighted to have my assessments and opinion challenged – I think almost, they should challenge me more." (L14)

Overall, surprisingly few consultants made any direct criticisms of the adversarial nature of contested final hearings.[15] This was not necessarily because they enjoyed the combative nature of such hearings, but because it was seen as a necessary and fundamental part of the process of testing the evidence and trying to get it right. In just the same way that many consultants did not want to see one view routinely imposed on the court, equally, in an effort to do their best and to contribute to the work of the court in the interests of children,

---

[15] Only one said he would like to see the issues removed from the courtroom altogether. Another recognised the need to examine the evidence closely but wanted a process that also 'healed'. A third consultant pointed out that not all consultants are good in the witness box because the 'gladiator' style did not necessarily suit them. It should be noted, however, that one selection criterion for this study – that respondents should still be accepting instructions in court work – may have influenced the range of findings in this area since arguably those most hostile to current practices may well no longer accept instructions. However, it could also be argued that one might have expected, given the comparative experiences tapped in this study, that the criticisms of other clinicians based on proceedings prior to the Children Act (e.g. King & Trowell, 1992) and those expressed in the early days of the Children Act (e.g. Wolkind, 1993) might have found a stronger representation in this sample.

cross-examination by a barrister was seen as an essential part of the process. In effect, it is their 'medicine': it may not necessarily taste good or always make them feel good – at least at the time – but it was perceived as an important feature of the family justice system and not one which could easily be replaced.

Thus, although court proceedings could generate a level of anxiety in consultants, these specialists thought that this was something with which they simply had to live. Indeed, in discussing this response, most consultants saw some benefits flowing from that situation. If they began to see it less seriously, for example if they felt they were getting what one termed as 'too slick' in presenting their views in court, and if giving oral evidence did not provoke some anxiety, it would be time to rethink their role. The knowledge that they could be heavily cross-examined about their work and the subsequent opinion was seen as a means of ensuring a strong self-critical perspective. But, equally important, it was also argued that if the courts became too uncritical of their views and if there was not an opportunity, in complex cases, for their work to be subjected to peer review, it would also be time for child psychiatrists to rethink their role and their contribution to proceedings between parents and the state, and, for some at least, it would be time for the psychiatrist to get out of the legal arena.

## The failures of the 1989 Children Act

Although consultants thought that proceedings following the 1989 Children Act have resulted in some substantial improvements to practices (see Box 3, above), views also indicate this is not a time for complacency. As Box 5 shows, consultants also expressed a number of

---

Box 5
*Criticisms of care proceedings under the Children Act 1989:*
*views and experiences of child psychiatrists*

- Proceedings were considered inferior compared with what was available within wardships proceedings.
- Inconsistency in court tribunals (i.e. different judges and magistrates) preparing cases for a final hearing.
- No assessment of the ability of the relevant CAMHS to provide the skills and time necessary for court work.
- Clinical expertise was sought too late in some cases.
- Failure to reconsider or debate the ethics of aspects of forensic work under the Act.
- Lack of a rigorous approach to expert evidence by some advocates and judges.

criticisms of current practices. Some of these criticisms arise directly from experiences during legal proceedings; others are related to the broader issues within child protection investigations and resources for family support services more generally.

Discussions indicated that, like guardians (Brophy *et al*, 1999*b*, p. 9), these consultants felt that many care applications brought under the 1989 Children Act would (prior to that Act) have been wardship proceedings. Consultants also compared what was possible under each and argued that under the Children Act the court lacked powers to oversee future important decisions in a child's life, for example ensuring a local authority secured any necessary therapeutic input for a child and carried out an agreed care plan. For these reasons, Children Act cases were viewed as inferior compared with what was considered possible under wardship proceedings.

Two points are relevant here. First, some of these views may be based on a somewhat idealised notion of what was actually achieved under wardship proceedings (for example, see Masson & Morton, 1989), and it remains the case that we do not know how, or indeed whether, most recommendations for treatment of children assessed during proceedings are carried forward. Second, recent research indicates that local authorities do not routinely change proposed care plans once a care order has been made (Hunt & Macleod, 1999). Thus, while some geographical variations may exist, this may be one of a number of popular myths in this field. But the issues that these consultants raise demonstrate at the least some important gaps in information in the system, as well as a lack of guarantee for follow-up work with very vulnerable children. Views also demonstrate a lack of feedback mechanism to these consultants with regard to the children they have assessed.

Consultants were also critical of the fact that judges cannot or do not reserve cases. Thus, during the preparation of a case a number of different judges can take directions hearings. Consultants felt this indicated a lack of continuity in case preparation, and if things went wrong they did not get picked up sufficiently early in proceedings. There are no national data on this issue, but there does appear to be some regional variation, with some courts attempting to ensure complex cases are listed before the same judge, and others finding this difficult if not impossible to achieve. However, it should be remembered that most cases involving experts (88%) are likely to start in the magistrates' family proceedings court, just over half of these (53%) are likely to be transferred, most (42%) are then finalised in a care centre/Principal Registry, but 11% are finalised in the High Court (Brophy *et al*, 1999*b*, table 4.3). Thus some discontinuity of tribunal is inevitable as cases are transferred between the different tiers of the family justice system. Moreover, in some courts, for example the Principal Registry of the Family Division, the volume of applications being heard and the limited number of judges available to hear applications make it unlikely that judges will be able to reserve cases; indeed, guardians serving this court have argued that 'you just don't know who you're going to get' (Brophy & Bates, 1999).[16] Thus, both child psychiatrists and guardians identify this as a failure in proceedings since the Children Act.

It should also be noted that research demonstrates that some of the most important decisions about the use and instruction of experts to assess children and parents are likely to be made in the magistrates' family proceedings courts (Bates & Brophy, 1996). Here, directions can be given by the family panel of magistrates, but if an application for leave to instruct an expert is uncontested, directions may well be made by a justices' clerk. Thus, in many cases that are transferred to a care centre (and thus come before a judge) it is likely that the judge will be relying on evidence that has been commissioned if not filed in the family proceedings court. The degree to which family panels in these courts are able to reserve cases is not known, but anecdotal evidence suggests that in some areas at least listing practices are making this possibility less likely, rather than more.

As demonstrated earlier, child psychiatrists also reported that increases in referrals in the context of legal proceedings have occurred alongside cutbacks in local CAMHS. Consultants argued that while substantial funds (from local authorities and from what was the Legal Aid Board) are being invested in assessments *within* legal proceedings, there are few or no resources for the treatment of children. Reduced resources in CAMHS clinics resulting in poor staffing levels and the loss of many multi-disciplinary teams has meant that where child psychiatrists have been able to offer at least some treatment after the proceedings, this has tended to be a less creative package than was previously possible. But consultants also reported that reductions in resources for preventive work have increased tensions for social workers trying to practise support in the community and the management of risk, and this has resulted in the late involvement of people with clinical skills in cases.[17]

As demonstrated in Chapter 4, a recurrent theme for some consultants working this field was that of moving from doctor to the family to

---

[16] This is also a criticism of notions of 'court control' made in the research of Hunt & Macleod (1998).

[17] There are no national data on this issue but available research from one study supports those views – relatively few cases demonstrate the involvement of CAMHS before the instigation of care proceedings (Bates & Brophy, 1996, table 25).

forensic expert for the court. Consultants felt this issue had been insufficiently addressed or understood by courts. It was argued that where a child psychiatrist had a clinical responsibility for a child and parent, and where that child subsequently became the subject of proceedings, there were some ethical issues that indicated that the psychiatrist, as the family's doctor, should not undertake the necessary forensic work. Consultants argued there had been a lack of recognition that the clinician's role is built on mutual trust between the clinician and the child and parents, and that this relationship was the result of *choice* on the part of parents and some children. As earlier discussions indicated, subsequent forensic work both with and without the informed consent of parents (and where applicable a child) raised ethical issues for psychiatrists, which they felt had not been adequately discussed or understood by courts or policy makers.

Finally, in listing their criticisms of practices following the Children Act, consultants returned to occasions when they thought their work and opinions had not been sufficiently challenged in court. At times they considered their work was treated with too much respect and they were not sufficiently challenged about their methods and the basis of their opinions. Moreover, some judges were also reported as being too ready to accept what experts say.

## Conclusions

As this chapter demonstrates, it would be a mistake to imagine that child psychiatrists working in this field are necessarily the passive recipients of policy initiatives. Some have been and continue to be involved in an ongoing debate about changes in both national and local policy. This chapter demonstrates two major themes arising from their experiences: first, the ethical issues that arise for some doctors who, on occasion, are expected to wear two hats; second, concerns about the way in which changes in the evidential process and in particular opportunities for peer review in complex cases raise some new and important questions about the relationship between 'law' and child welfare knowledge discourses.

Responses indicate that an important clinical agenda is emerging from clinicians undertaking assessments within child protection litigation – albeit perhaps a somewhat uncoordinated agenda because of the lack of a national professional forum within which child psychiatrists can discuss and develop their work in this field. Nevertheless, these consultants were clear about the contribution of their skills and disciplines (both child psychiatry and psychology) to the questions posed by child care law, and ready to challenge misunderstandings about hard and soft evidence, and to educate courts and advocates in this field.

While there were areas of agreement and clear support for changes to many practices and procedures regarding the use and work of expert evidence following the Children Act, there were areas of criticism. Many of the issues raised have also been identified by other professionals working in the family justice system. Lack of resources for Children Act proceedings permeated much of this discussion. Some consultants outlined ethical concerns that need to be discussed by the profession as a whole. While these child psychiatrists wholly accepted a duty to the court and not to instructing parties, they also maintained an independent ethical duty of care to the child.

This duty has several ramifications. It moved some experts on occasion to go beyond, challenge or change instructions, and to criticise court practices and procedures. Equally, an ethical duty of care to the child led some clinicians to argue that it may well be unethical for child psychiatrists to undertake assessments and make treatment recommendations that they, as doctors, could not take forward. This issue may be a point of tension between those still working in the NHS and those who are retired and thus both an institutional but also a generational issue. Ethical concerns also arose because of the frequent use of child psychiatrists at the point of crisis in many children's lives but with little resources for early involvement or post-court follow-up treatment.

Ethical concerns also emerged in discussions about recent legal policy initiatives to deal with potentially competing expert evidence. A central concern here was with lack of understanding on the part of courts and policy makers about the nature of child welfare knowledge and the scientific process. As the training and experience of these clinicians demonstrate, competing paradigms are the lifeblood of science and central to the development of knowledge in this field. While 'law' may prefer to see child welfare knowledge as a unitary category, that model is not supported by scientists in general, or by the consultants in this study. This is *not* to say that there is resistance to improving the quality of court work or to attempts to narrow down real differences between experts, for example in pre-trial meetings. Despite some practical problems with some meetings, they have in principle been welcomed and seen as worthwhile. However, where consultants saw practices as trying to eliminate the possibility of *any* disagreement, this posed some ethical questions as to the real role and function of the psychiatrist in the legal arena.

On the whole, this sample expressed relatively little concern about the clinicians who are viewed as 'hired guns' or 'rubber stamps' in this field, and this may be a decreasing problem in Children Act proceedings. Few of the interviewees initially saw themselves in this light. But they also outlined how a reputation in this relatively small field can be acquired: on the basis of a pattern of preferred instructing parties, or types of referral, past research reputation, a specialist clinical practice and word of mouth. It would also be naive to suggest that instructing parties do not, on occasion, seek out certain experts on a given criterion. Most of these experts tried to emphasise the issue of balance and neutrality in their work. However, they were candid and realistic. Most of the national experts thought they were probably identified with particular views; fewer clinicians working in local services thought they might be, but they could see how reputations developed despite their own beliefs about their views and practices.

# 6 Child psychiatrists and the family justice system: a multi-disciplinary, multi-agency agenda

## *Introduction*

This study suggests that, at the end of the 1990s, after almost a decade of Children Act proceedings, the use of child psychiatrists within child protection litigation required a radical review. Practices have grown out of an often uncoordinated and fragmented response to demands for increasingly sophisticated clinical expertise, as 'law' attempted to move further towards more transparent and evidence-based decision making in complex cases of child abuse and neglect.

Much of this (forensic) work evolved out of private practice and current modes of provision are a legacy of the 1948 settlement of consultants' contracts (see below). Further changes proposed for these contracts since the completion of this study make even it more imperative that this issue remains on the legal, political and clinical agenda. NHS reforms (Department of Health, 2000) indicate a review of existing consultants' contracts aimed at increasing the number of contracted NHS sessions (from five to seven) (para. 8.23) while reducing dramatically the time available for other (non-NHS) work. Moreover, the aim is for newly qualified consultants to be contracted to work *exclusively* for the NHS perhaps for the first seven years of their career.[1] Both these changes, if instigated, are likely to have considerable implications for the future of work in the public law arena.

---

[1] Para 8.24 of the *NHS Plan* (Department of Health, 2000) states "newly qualified consultants will be contracted to work exclusively for the NHS for perhaps the first

There is therefore a need to articulate a clear statement of policy aims and service development plans in this field, along with a statement of ethics that takes into account the new landscape identified by these and other clinicians working in the family justice system.

The study identified some regional variations in practices and views about appropriate tasks and functions of child psychiatrists in this field. There are indications of high-quality work by clinicians who are clearly very committed to this type of work. Despite lack of attention by policy makers to the fact that few clinicians appeared to be contracted to undertake this work or to the lack of resources and training for it within many CAMHS, the clinicians in this study at least responded positively to much of the new agenda that 'the law' set them. However, there are also examples of arrogance and an imperviousness to the skills of other professionals, for example overriding instructions without consultation, being unaware of the responsibilities and skills of social workers, exhibiting poor skills with some parents, perceiving themselves as taking control rather than as team players in a process and, on occasion, taking on a judicial function.

Some problems with the provision of a service are historical in origin; others result from a lack of lead from government in the early days of the Act. This policy lacuna contributed to an already fragmented response to local need from many hard-pressed local services. For example, research indicates little evidence of a clinical input to cases before the instigation of legal proceedings and few real opportunities for continuity of clinical input once proceedings are completed. Other problems, however, arose from idiosyncratic or poor practices by individual experts and/or instructing parties.

This final chapter therefore considers two themes. First, the current model of provision of CAMHS for courts is considered along with the implications for training, earlier collaborative work between agencies, service renewal issues (once the current generation of experts fully retire) and questions of appropriate ethics and accountability within services. Second, findings from the study on the tasks undertaken by child psychiatrists are discussed along with implications for theoretical debates about the relationship between child welfare knowledge and legal discourses in the twenty-first century.

---

seven years of their career, providing eight fixed sessions, and more of the service delivery out of hours ... the right to undertake private practice will depend on fulfilling job plan and NHS service requirements including satisfactory appraisals. If agreement cannot be secured to these changes, the Government will look to introduce a new specialist grade for newly qualified specialists to secure similar objectives."

## *Service provision for the twenty-first century*

### 'Good enough' services to assess 'good enough' parenting: within or without the NHS?

Few professionals could have anticipated the level of demand that care proceedings have generated for specialist input from child psychiatrists. Nevertheless, the study indicates a range of highly sensitive questions that continue to require attention by central government and by a range of professional bodies. Central concerns, such as the need to develop a national framework, standards and a timeframe for service delivery and methods of accountability[2] and training require a concerted programme and investment. A major and unavoidable question arising from this study is whether public law work should remain largely outside mainstream NHS clinical practice. It is hard to find a child-focused justification for it remaining so. While practices remain largely outside of mainstream NHS work, it will be difficult, if not impossible, to establish:

(a) accountability for the service;
(b) universal training standards;
(c) responsibility for ensuring the input of a new generation of experts;
(d) clinical continuity for some children.

When the proposed changes to consultants' contracts are included in this equation and thus a reduction if not elimination of the extra-contractual/private time in which this work is currently undertaken, the case for the inclusion of public law work within the NHS seems irrefutable.

In addition, under current conditions it is not easy to compare costs for these services[3] or to determine whether they represent the best value for money. Nor is it clear how 'value' should be measured. This is a nettle that neither local health services nor other bodies (e.g. local and central government) have been willing to grasp. But as the NHS Health Advisory Service (1995, p. 2) argued in relation to CAMHS

---

[2] Or 'clinical governance', as it is increasingly called within the NHS.
[3] For example, a register of experts produced by one GALRO panel indicated that child psychiatrists have a range of hourly fees (from £90 to £170 per hour) and methods of charging (e.g. some differentiate costs between assessment time, court time, travelling time and waiting time, others charge a flat hourly rate, others quote an inclusive figure, etc.). Changes to the funding of cases by the Community Legal Service (see note 4 below) are likely to bring some uniformity to this field if not to the hourly rates charged.

generally, ad hoc responses to need are expensive and they present considerable problems to planning strategies. Yet substantial government-funded research (e.g. Bates & Brophy, 1996; Hunt & Macleod, 1998; Brophy *et al*, 1999*b*) now demonstrates that the needs of courts and families for specialist assessments can no longer be described as ad hoc and that they have indeed suffered from a lack of planning, investment and control.

In one very real sense it has been 'law' rather than 'health' that has driven this issue. Developments demonstrate there is little space or motivation for turning back. There is, of course, room for improvement, for example in the quality and delivery of these services and for ensuring they are appropriately used. But the interdisciplinary nature of family law *practice* – and thus the use of specialist expertise – is no longer debatable, as Mr Justice Wall (1995) argued:

> "Let there be no mistake about this. The judges of the [Family] Division readily acknowledge that Family Law is multi-disciplinary. Indeed the proposition is axiomatic, particularly in the field of child protection."

The provision of a multi-disciplinary *service*, however, remains problematic, at least so far as CAMHS are concerned. Central questions remain about responsibility for providing, maintaining, reviewing and renewing these services. This is a rather curious situation in the UK, where other services, such as health and social care, are increasingly subject to the implementation of quality standards, clinical governance, best-value initiatives and inspection and review. But while the internal market in the NHS has largely been abolished, the view of the UK government appears to remain that these very specific health services – aimed to assist complex decision making in disputes between families and the state – should remain largely extra-contractual and thus outside of the NHS, with the purchaser of the service meeting the direct costs.[4]

In these circumstances much work is likely to remain largely unregulated and the establishment of nationally agreed standards is rendered difficult because many clinicians are not responsible to an NHS trust or the Department of Health for the quality of their public law work. Equally, except where the professional parties simply avoid

---

[4] All the more curious because, in practice, the majority of the costs for expert witnesses in public law proceedings are met from the public purse. In the case of local authority instructions, costs are met, in part, from local taxation. In the case of instructions from guardians and most parents, costs are now met by the Legal Services Commission – since April 2000, the Commission has managed the Community Legal Service Fund (CLS), which replaced the Legal Aid Board.

reappointing child psychiatrists whose work they consider substandard or where a judge comments adversely on the report or evidence of a particular expert, we have no way of knowing, as one standard of appraisal, "whether these services are considered useful by the population they serve" (NHS Health Advisory Service, 1995, p. 3) – there is no means of quality control.

Those within and outside child psychiatry who view this area of forensic work with some cynicism have tended to argue that because it is a highly lucrative field of work for individuals it is very unlikely that support for any changes will come from within the profession. That view is not supported by this research. Many of the child psychiatrists in this study argued that it was time to rethink this service, based on developments and experiences following the Children Act 1989.

This is not, however, an easy area of health provision to change, in part because, historically, it has been located under the umbrella of forensic services. As indicated above, the extra-contractual nature of much of this work lies in the post-war development of the NHS and the exclusion of certain categories of work from mainstream (category 1) NHS work.[5] When this occurred, medico-legal work was a relatively minor service and child protection work within it largely insignificant. However, the conditions that precipitated the exclusion of this type of work from mainstream NHS practice cannot be compared with the social and economic conditions, medical expertise and policy approaches to child abuse and neglect that exist at the start of the twenty-first century. The way in which we attempt to deal with child maltreatment by parents bears no comparison with attitudes to child abuse in the 1950s. Many of the questions that are now posed by 'law' (see Fig. 1, p. 9), for example with regard to allegations of sexual, physical and emotional abuse, and the knowledge base and measures that are necessary demand the skills and expertise of health professionals. This is part of the process of making evidence-based decisions about children's lives, where the aim is to assist local authorities and courts in making what, in practice, is often the least detrimental alternative for children, many of whom have already suffered substantial maltreatment.

**The need for more effective collaboration between health and social services but also independent services**

Certain issues require the attention of central government in order to secure a better national framework for the delivery of CAMHS for

---

[5] This history is briefly discussed by Brophy *et al* (1999*a*, p. 87) but it is outlined in more detail by Digby (1989, p. 60) and Webster (1988, p. 80).

children within public law proceedings. Research in the 1990s (e.g. Bates & Brophy, 1996; Brophy *et al*, 1999*b*) revealed that too often crisis intervention rather than coherent planning characterised the input of CAMHS into child protection work. The views and experiences of clinicians in this study provide some of the major reasons underlying that approach. While a framework for pre-court collaboration between health and social services exists under section 27 of the Children Act 1989,[6] resources for this work did not. There were several indications that many local authorities have not achieved much success in trying to use section 27 to obtain the help of health authorities (as they were then called) in obtaining specialist assessments. Indeed, section 27 seems generally to be regarded by social workers, guardians and child psychiatrists as ineffective because it has no teeth: a local authority can request help but there is no statutory duty on health services to comply.

However, policy climates seldom stand still. Since the completion of this study there have been a number of initiatives aimed at improving collaboration between local NHS trusts and local authorities, most notably social services departments. Further research is necessary to identify whether any of the new government initiatives aimed at breaking down the 'Berlin Wall' between agencies (Dobson, 1997) have been successful. There is some *potential* for new localised funding strategies for child protection work, for example under the Quality Protects programme for local authorities and from the new money (£84 million)

---

[6] Section 27 (cooperation between authorities) authorises a local authority to request the help of another authority or person specified in section 27(3), which includes any health authority (as these were called at that time). An authority whose help is so requested "shall comply with the request if it is compatible with their own statutory duties and obligations and does not unduly prejudice the discharge of any of their functions." In other words, it is not a statutory duty to comply with a request and, as this study identifies, in the light of greatly reduced resources and a paucity of adequately experienced and trained staff, it is likely that many health authorities would be unable or unwilling to comply with such a request.

[7] Quality Protects is a three-year government programme designed to change the management and delivery of social services for children in England and Wales. All local authorities were required to submit a management action plan to the Department of Health by the end of January 1999. Under these plans a local authority could choose to earmark some of the available new money to purchase clinical services to provide assessments and support social workers in child protection cases. There is no information about how many local authorities opted to do this and there remain problems with finding appropriately skilled people and with developing criteria with which to assess work. Equally, CAMHS could use some of the additional £84 million child mental health grant to develop services in this field – although this money is intended to expand general clinical services and improve geographical coverage.

awarded to CAMHS.[7] But despite evidence-based research and pressures from some consultant child psychiatrists, none of this new money is *mandated* to improve services for child protection litigation. Thus, any positive developments in this field will once again be down to local choice.

It is therefore especially important to ascertain whether collaboration and more effective joint working between health and social care agencies are actually being achieved, and whether this has an identifiable impact on the quality and quantity of clinical pre-court work being undertaken with families. It is especially important to investigate these issues given the funding traditions and long-standing organisational, cultural and professional differences identified in this study.[8] However, an improved multi-agency approach between local authorities and child health services prior to and within legal proceedings is only one part of the equation. The services of clinicians who are independent of the local authority must also be available to parents and to guardians as independent representatives of children.

### Reluctant clinicians: bringing in the silent majority?

Consultants in this study argued that public law work is some of the best and most important they can do, but this area of work has not appealed to many child psychiatrists. Secondary sources identify several reasons for this[9] and, as Table 10 shows, lack of training, experience and confidence are key issues in five primary areas of concern.

Table 10 also shows that there are some common views between clinicians who do this work and those who have refused: both groups identify work overload in general clinical practice and both groups express concerns about the ethical issues the work can generate. Moreover, developments in child protection litigation following the Children Act 1989 may well have increased the element of exclusivity that attaches to this work, for example by extending and tightening the responsibilities of experts, by attempting the timetabling of their reports and by insisting on pre-trial meetings in the case of conflicting expert opinion. These developments may have made the choice of

---

[8] Of some concern is the growth in small, unregulated private businesses set up solely to respond to the shortfall in skills and staff availability within local NHS clinical provision. Anecdotal evidence from appraisals of some of this work suggests some further investigation may be necessary.

[9] In a national random survey of guardians they were asked a range of questions about any difficulties they had experienced in finding experts able and willing to accept instructions, actual failures to appoint, and about the reasons for clinicians being unwilling to work in this field (Brophy *et al*, 1999*b*).

TABLE 10
*Reasons why child psychiatrists are unwilling to accept instructions within public law proceedings*

| Type of reason | Specific example |
| --- | --- |
| Lack of time | General clinical overload and thus a reluctance to waste time in court |
| Ethical issues | Role conflict between therapeutic and forensic work |
| Anxieties about legal methods | Reluctance to submit to cross-examination in contested hearings, objections to being 'grilled' in court, unwillingness to open work to criticism or peer review |
| Lack of appropriate training and experience | Anxiety provoked by the idea of court work |
| Doubts about the validity of assessments for courts | The psychiatrist can often only state the obvious and there is therefore little professional interest in this category of work |

Source: Brophy *et al* (1999*b*, p. 16).

whether to do any of this type of work less rather than more likely for clinicians with no real experience of it (both newly qualified and established clinicians).

At the end of the 1990s, two issues forced something of a backlash. Evidence of an absence of real opportunities for specialist registrars to acquire the relevant experience became apparent, and research evidence pointed towards not only a current shortfall of willing and able child psychiatrists but also a projected and even more serious shortfall in the next generation of child psychiatrists who may be willing and *acceptable* as expert witnesses in the twenty-first century.

Since the completion of this study, some training initiatives have sought to address these issues. First, reviews of specialist training in the preparation of clinicians for consultant status demonstrated that it has been difficult for specialist registrars to gain experience of giving evidence-in-chief. Research demonstrates that this has primarily been because advocates and guardians have been unwilling to appoint experts below consultant status (Brophy *et al*, 1999*b*, p. 17). Thus, it has been difficult, if not impossible, for clinicians to complete one of the three tasks necessary to demonstrate core experience in forensic child protection work. Routine review of training has subsequently resulted in a change to guidance in this field by the Child and Adolescent Psychiatry Specialist Advisory Committee (1999). This has been amended – in the short term at least – to allow clinicians to qualify for consultant status where they can demonstrate *attendance* at court hearings and *observation* of an experienced child psychiatrist giving evidence and, where possible, giving evidence in court with a trainer present.

Second, the possibilities for specialist registrars to gain the necessary experience in observing court proceedings has been increased by recent initiatives from the President's Interdisciplinary Family Law Committee. In order to try to encourage more child psychiatrists at specialist registrar level to work in the family justice system, judges have been encouraged to develop local initiatives to allow these clinicians to spend time sitting in with judges to gain observational experience of court proceedings.

Entering this field nevertheless holds a number of professional anxieties and undeniable risks for newcomers in a profession with a very strong hierarchical tradition. For example, specialist registrars are unlikely to be entirely at ease giving a second opinion on the work of a more senior colleague: some may well be at least initially uncomfortable to have their opinions pitched against consultants with a national or international reputation.[10] There may also be concerns about the implications for future career prospects in a profession where an individual consultant can exert considerable power in terms of the promotion ladder.

It is also the case that some new training initiatives need to focus on increasing the participation of existing consultants. This is a complex area, where multi-disciplinary discussions about post-qualification training for all professionals in the family justice system are in their infancy. For many clinicians undertaking this work, ongoing training has been elective rather than mandatory. This issue needs to be confronted with regard to both changes to core training programmes for newcomers (see above) and future training for existing consultants. The study points to a need for post-qualification interdisciplinary training that incorporates a wider understanding of the core training and skills across all the professional groups involved in child protection litigation. At the time of the study there had been little or no consideration of a common core curriculum aimed at achieving an agreed national standard of core knowledge and practices across available courses. Thus, available post-qualification training in this field for all professional groups has been somewhat fragmented and uncoordinated. In the absence of mandatory interdisciplinary training based on a system of accreditation, mutual misunderstandings, criticisms, mistrust and examples of poor interdisciplinary and inter-agency practice are likely to continue.

---

[10] And the evidence indicates that parties are generally not willing to risk instructing psychiatrists who are less senior and arguably less experienced than the consultant instructed by a local authority (Brophy & Bates, 1998).

There are also some inescapable dilemmas and tensions here within and between clinical cultures and the needs of 'the law' and the culture of courts. The concerns and career structures of registrars outlined above cannot be overlooked, but nor can their need for hands-on experience. But the traditional culture of courts in this field is also problematic. As outlined in the Introduction, historically, the status and experience of an expert witness have provided fertile ground for advocates testing their advocacy skills, where one aim has been to undermine an expert's credibility in part on the basis of a lack of status and experience. If clinicians below consultant status are to be instructed, in the short term at least judges may have to exert more control during cross-examination to ensure advocates do not indulge in personal attacks and attempts to humiliate witnesses.

This is *not*, however, an argument for a less rigorous testing of the *evidence* – quite the contrary – but some advocates will need to change traditional and arguably outmoded practices so far as Children Act cases are concerned, and specialist registrars must have some training and courtroom experience if this is to be achieved. Advocates and guardians will need to be assured of the training and ability of clinicians new to the field. Research demonstrates this has not been an area where they are willing to take risks – and this is likely to be increasingly the case if pressures towards joint instructions continue. Guardians rightly demand the best expertise for some of the most vulnerable children in society, who have often already been seriously failed by adults. Thus, it is the responsibility of policy makers and trainers to ensure training and competence standards are met. In particular, parental abuse should not be followed by a new form of system abuse, in which inexperienced clinicians fail children through a lack of appropriate training, support and experience.

### Contemporary ethics for working in the child protection arena

Ethical concerns and dilemmas for the child psychiatrist in the legal arena appeared at a number of points in discussions. These clinicians (and others – see below) pointed to the need for a much wider debate of a number of concerns in the light of contemporary development – medical ethics *per se* were not necessarily always seen as appropriate to or sufficient for the task. For example, wider debate is required about:

    (a)  the ethics of moving from a treatment to a forensic brief;
    (b)  the ethics covering assessments for courts;
    (c)  ethical issues and debates raised in other jurisdictions;
    (d)  the ethics appropriate for a seamless system of provision for children;

(e) the ethical implications for the psychiatric profession of a single, jointly appointed expert.

Some of the child psychiatrists in this study highlighted the ethical concerns that arose for them when they were asked to move from a treatment-based relationship with children and parents to a forensic exercise for the purposes of legal proceedings. They felt this issue had not been fully understood or appreciated by some local authorities or courts. Nor, it seems, has this ethical concern been much discussed by clinicians themselves (e.g. in professional journals) in the UK.

Some clinicians view the work that they do for courts as having a therapeutic role in itself (e.g. Sturge, 1992; Tufnell, 1993b). Sturge, for example, argued that Children Act cases offer the potential for positive intervention as a means to further the child's interests. Thus, report writing for courts is seen as inseparable from the therapeutic intervention and it is not therefore viewed as merely procedural. In other jurisdictions, however, some doubt has been cast on whether this perspective – which relies on general medical ethics – is appropriate for forensic work (see below).

Professional concerns about the ethics of forensic work by psychiatrists and psychologists are more evident in other jurisdictions. For example, several clinicians in North America have highlighted an absence of theoretical and ethical debate in forensic psychiatry generally – despite the fact that the Academy of Psychiatry and the Law has existed in North America for some 30 years (Rappeport, 1999). Looking at issues of professional accountability of the expert witness in the Family Court in New Zealand, Murfitt (2000) highlighted some of the tensions that have arisen between the professional body for psychologists and the Family Court with regard to appropriate ethics for assessments within litigation (as opposed to ethics covering therapeutic treatment), and disciplinary procedures.

Recent debates (e.g. Simon & Wettstein, 1997; Appelbaum, 1997; O'Brien, 1998) resulted from an assertion that forensic psychiatrists lack clear guidelines about what is ethical with respect to their professional activities in the legal arena and, therefore, they should stay out of the courtroom. O'Brien (1998) concurred that this issue has been inadequately addressed by psychiatrists in Australia. He argued that there should be a greater emphasis on developing integrated community-based forensic services but with leadership coming from within the profession rather than being driven by government. Appelbaum (1997), writing in North America, argued that forensic psychiatry cannot simply reply on general medical ethics embedded in the doctor–patient relationship, since this is absent from the forensic setting. Like some consultants in this study, Appelbaum argues that any endeavours to retain a residuum of the doctor–patient relationship and its ethical principles are likely to result in what is referred to as 'double agency'.

The future of forensic services for family courts is neither settled nor safe. But, as some of the child psychiatrists in this study argued, if, in looking at future policy, one starts with the needs of highly vulnerable children rather than trying to work within the institutional and structural legacies of a post-war economy, one might construct a very different approach and service. As a policy objective, for example, a seamless service – one that can provide early assessment and treatment, assessments for legal proceedings where necessary and, where appropriate, follow-up treatment for children – has a number of real benefits, not least of which is continuity of care and support for a child.

However, this is a very complex issue; while some consultants wanted to be able to provide a seamless and more holistic service, ethical issues within this approach also require wider debate. As this study found, some consultants were very protective of the rights and feelings of parents in this area. For some parents, the move from a treatment focus to a forensic role by their doctors raised questions, for example concerning the degree to which the clinician could and would be seen to be completely independent of the local authority instigating proceedings. This issue was also of concern to guardians (Brophy & Bates, 1999).[11] These concerns and dilemmas must be to the forefront when considering the development of a seamless service. It must be borne in mind, for example, that it is likely such a service would make a substantial contribution to a local authority's care plan, which would form part of a local authority's evidence. Thus, some flexibility would need to be retained in attempts to provide more holistic CAMHS in order for services to hold the confidence of both parents and guardians.

## *The tasks of the child psychiatrist: legal and welfare discourses*

### Competing discourses

Findings indicated that the process of interpretation of behaviour, past events and existing and future risks, and the transformation of what are essentially welfare questions into a series of choices on which

---

[11] For example, some guardians have argued that in these circumstances (i.e. where it is proposed to instruct an expert within proceedings who had a prior treatment-based relationship with a family), there were strong arguments for considering a change of expert for the purposes of litigation.

a court *sometimes* has to make a contested decision, is more complex than previously suggested. Where previously 'law' may have been experienced as oversimplifying problems and behaviours in order to reduce them to simple legal categories and ultimately dominating welfare discourses, there are now indications that this relationship is changing. Evidence from this study indicates that child welfare specialists with experience of cases both before and after implementation of the Children Act do not necessarily experience current proceedings in this way.

As Chapter 3 demonstrated, in the light of the range of questions posed by 'law', parties generally required a package from these child welfare experts. This package covered information about current or previous harm, future risks and parents' ability and willingness to change. That agenda is of course largely set by the threshold criteria[12] and thus the demands of law, but these demands are for a range of health-based information. This is *not* to say that this evidence is free from controversy. Rather, that, in principle at least, new procedures were part of an attempt at evidence-based and more accountable practices. The aim was for more transparency in cases, and the move from largely oral to written evidence, the timetabling of evidence and the loss of professional privilege have all been powerful changes in making parties more accountable for their actions. But the structure of the significant harm criteria, in principle, also aimed to make experts more accountable for their opinions and the assessment framework on which these are based.

There is evidence, for example with regard to both how cases are defined and questions posed and how consultants present and defend their field of knowledge in court, which indicates that the consultants in this study, at least, were likely to confront and, if necessary, override certain limitations that 'the law' may seek to impose on their work. These responses suggest that the relationship between the two discourses, the law and child welfare knowledge, is now a more interactive, multi-dimensional process than was previously apparent. In this process, the experts (the purveyors of child welfare knowledge) do not *necessarily* find their knowledge transformed or their concerns and judgements subordinated to the perceived needs and legal categories imposed by 'law'. Rather, in Children Act proceedings, practices indicated that a process of negotiation can take place in which child welfare specialists perceive they are making considerable

---

[12] Section 31(2) of the Children Act 1989 – see Fig. 1, p. 9, but also section 1(5), whereby the court must also consider whether making the order would be better for the child than making any other order or no order at all.

progress at a number of levels. And while 'the law' is having to learn that child welfare knowledge does not offer absolute 'truths', it is also the case that experts are having to justify and define more clearly their own activities and the procedures they apply for validating their knowledge base – and that is absolutely appropriate. Most clinicians in this study appeared comfortable with that challenge, but it is arguably a relatively new experience for some.

Moreover, given an ongoing lack of resources for real investment in the family justice system and in the necessary supporting health services on which it is heavily dependent, it is suggested that, in practice, both arenas are subordinated to a primary agenda of central government: that of reducing expenditure on legal services.

**Risk assessment – the clinical response**

The clinical assessment of future risk is now a central part of child protection litigation. Although research does not support the view that there is a multiplicity of experts in most cases all addressing the same issue (Bates & Brophy, 1996; Hunt & Macleod, 1998; Brophy *et al*, 1999*b*), it is important that the complexity of a clinical assessment of risk as outlined by consultants in this study is understood. A central message is that the cases referred to these consultants are usually very complex – several factors and their *interrelationship* need to be assessed – and in these circumstances an adequate risk assessment can rarely be done by one person only. This is a principle for practice laid down by the Royal College of Psychiatrists' Special Working Party on Clinical Assessment and Management of Risk (1996).

In many cases involving current harm and the assessment and possibilities for the management of future risks, reports were based on a synthesis of clinical and other information. For example, in cases of alleged sexual or physical abuse, consultants did not work in isolation of the views of other professionals. Research shows that there is generally a sequence to the evidence-gathering process in these cases. Certain types of medical evidence (e.g. reports from paediatricians, paediatric radiologists or neurologists) are usually sought and filed first. Mental health evidence then follows (Bates & Brophy, 1996). Thus, following leave of the court for psychiatric family assessments and for disclosure of existing reports,[13] child psychiatrists usually have a range of information and opinions from other professionals. As

---

[13] That is, permission of the court for the party(ies) instructing the expert to disclose to that expert documents (reports and statements) already filed in a case.

Chapter 3 identifies, in these complex cases consultants argued that the contribution of the child psychiatrist was to add their own assessment – especially about future needs and options – and offer the court a reasonably reliable prognosis about the future.

Contrary to much received wisdom, not all applications for care orders are likely to include issues of physical or sexual abuse. Many cases are likely to be concerned with allegations of neglect and the alleged failure of parents to meet a child's physical, emotional and psychological needs, the measurement of that failure and its impact on the child.[14] In many cases it is likely there will be multiple issues and concerns about the level of care and protection provided for a child. There may, for example, also be concerns about drug abuse or about the impact of adult mental health problems or personality disorders, physical disability, an inappropriate partner and male violence on a child.[15] A multiplicity of concerns increases the complexity of the assessment exercise and this is especially so where there are concerns about more than one child in a family. Pulling together complex issues, assessing future risk and deciding a parent's capacity for change, bearing in mind a child's timescale[16], this exercise and the analysis and synthesis of information often demand clinical skills.

In many cases professionals will be concerned about whether a child has suffered emotional abuse or is likely to do so if a parent's behaviour does not change. Psychiatrists have argued that a diagnosis of emotional abuse is a complex exercise and prognosis in such cases is also likely to require particular skills and clinical training, and thus likely to fall within the remit of the child psychiatrist (Jones, 1991; Kaplan & Thompson, 1995).

## Clinical expertise and social work expertise

As Chapter 3 demonstrates, parties usually look to these clinicians to supply a package of information and, as Box 3 illustrates, the package that consultants argued they could offer in terms of 'added value' to

---

[14] Research based in one local authority (five family proceedings courts, one care centre, 114 children) found that just under two-thirds of cases did not contain allegations of sexual or physical abuse (Bates & Brophy, 1996, tables 12 and 13).
[15] And many applications are likely to cite lack of parental cooperation with a local authority as one of the reasons for court proceedings. Bates & Brophy (1996) note this was one of a number of reasons in some 62% of applications.
[16] And these will be set by a child's response to maltreatment, the child's age and emotional and developmental needs, etc. Thus, the time frame is set by the needs of the child and not those of the parents.

proceedings was, in principle, impressive. But further research is necessary. One of the issues this study sought to elucidate from experts was their definition of their skills and contributions to proceedings. Much of that material requires further empirical verification, that is, research that tests whether they do, in practice, cover a multi-disciplinary framework (including biological, psychological, emotional and social perspectives) and draw on a range of theories and techniques to judge, for example, the potential for change in parents who frequently have multiple pressures and problems.

We now know how 'added value' is constructed, at least by clinicians, but the question, forcefully put by one consultant, remains: "Do we really know our stuff in this field, is it clearly demonstrated in our work?" To address this question it was first necessary to unpack the product in order to provide a baseline. It should be remembered that the indications are that most consultants do not work in multi-disciplinary teams for the purposes of public law referrals. Thus, a great deal of work and opinion rest in the hands of one practitioner. Equally, as Table 3 shows, some will see a family on one occasion only. This snapshot approach has been criticised by guardians as usually insufficient (Brophy & Bates, 1998). As Table 7 suggests, there is a substantial amount of information to be obtained in one interview. Moreover, variation in the number of appointments different child psychiatrists generally undertake with families requires further investigation. This study suggests a possible link between the number of appointments and the institutional and contractual base, with local experts in this study appearing to spend more time with families than national experts (see Table 2). If these data do demonstrate a national trend, the reasons and the costs and benefits of this variation require exploration.

There is also a need to reassess and make more transparent the training and expertise of social workers in the field of child protection.[17] This is a complex area because, as the research indicates, there is a wide variation in skills and little available information on the distribution of postgraduate social workers across local authorities. Consultants reported that some social workers had provided some excellent pre-clinical assessments. They were also seen as having very specific and important skills, for example being able to identify risk and potential

---

[17] Since the completion of this study, social work training in England and Wales has undergone review. It has long been a contention of many people working in this particular field that social work should be a graduate profession and those undertaking child protection work should have additional postgraduate training. A government green paper addressing proposed reforms to social work training was due in the summer of 2000. Indications are that it will recommend a three-year degree course for all those wishing to enter this field.

risk. Moreover, social workers also provided information on practical issues such as rehousing, parenting skills, social networks and social support for parents. But a claim to specialist expertise in this field, that is, expertise beyond skills of a somewhat practical nature and being able to identify 'a concern' and potential risk in families, requires attention, clarification and wider publicity and understanding by other professionals.

This issue is clearly controversial. Some writers have asked whether, given the increase in the use of experts for child and family assessments, social workers retain claims to any clinical expertise in family work.[18] The consultants in this study argued that they 'added value' to proceedings in terms of the range and depth of clinical training and experience undertaken. And clearly, as Box 2 demonstrates, much of this training and expertise is highly specialist. But we did not examine or compare the training of child psychiatrists, for example in child development and attachment theory, with that likely to have been undertaken by a senior social worker with some post-qualification training. Once new proposals for core training in both professions are clearer, clarification and perhaps some long-term improvements in both fields can be anticipated.

However, what would also be productive for the family justice system would be the introduction of some mandatory, interdisciplinary post-qualification training modules to be undertaken by all professionals wishing to work in this increasingly specialised field. The development of appropriate modules would be an exciting challenge. It would inevitably have to address and test knowledge in, for example, child development and the attachment needs of children, assessing a parent or carer's willingness and capacity to provide appropriate care and protection, and mechanisms for addressing a parent's capacity for change in an acceptable time span, and so on. In so doing, such an exercise would also *have* to identify the boundaries and inevitable overlap of certain claims to knowledge and expertise.

---

[18] This question is not new, nor is it limited to the increased use of mental health experts in care proceedings. For example, Hopkins (1996, p. 29) argued that a loss of claims to any clinical expertise is in part due to the introduction of theoretical models in social work training that reframed problems experienced by clients as a response to present problems, rather than past circumstances. Others (e.g. Cooper *et al*, 1995; Hallett, 1996; Otway, 1996; Parton, 1996; Robinson, 1996) raised questions about the way in which 'the law', with its emphasis on assessment and evidence, is overdetermining contemporary social work practice with children and families. This debate is complex and beyond the boundaries of this book, but the 'added value' that consultants in this study argued they brought and evidence of the lack of comprehensive social work assessments before some proceedings do raise questions about why social work assessments are not being undertaken and also why local consultants are not involved earlier in some cases.

In addition, knowledge of the child protection and family support system as a whole would need to form an essential part of a post-qualification curriculum. Thus, parties and courts could be assured that a clinician who had attended such a course would fully understand the tasks and responsibilities of local authorities, the role of the social worker and what, for example, should have been covered in a social worker's assessment and the weight that should therefore be accorded to a social worker's opinion.

There is one further point in this context that needs to be reiterated. To consultants' own views of their 'added value' to proceedings and their range of specialist training and experience must be added the extra cachet of status that these specialists have by virtue of being medically trained. This brings a largely unspoken, but ever present, power and authority to their views. Doctors, particularly consultants, are accorded high socio-economic status in most Western European societies. That background gives most consultants considerable confidence and an expectation of trust, respect and, at times, deference in society.

Some consultants, however, are becoming increasingly critical of the impact of these issues on their work in some courts. This is not, as previously argued, because they have been subjected to humiliating cross-examination, but rather that their work has sometimes not been subjected to a sufficiently rigorous scrutiny. In some courts at least, reputation and high social status have impeded critical appraisal of clinical evidence and opinion. Certain clinicians perceived this as a dangerous trend, for individual experts, for child psychiatry as a discipline, and for children and the courts.

## Clinicians' responses to the new legal agenda

As Chapter 4 demonstrates, for the most part changes to the work of experts instigated by a new legal agenda have been welcomed by these child psychiatrists. Improving instructions to experts has formed a central part of this agenda and three issues are apparent.

First, most consultants were clear that their duty in care proceedings was to assist the court and not further the cause of an instructing party. Nevertheless (and somewhat paradoxically), consultants clearly had preferences and most preferred instructions from the guardian, or, as one consultant described it, "being on the side of the angels".

So far as the position of parents is concerned, given that one of the aims of the Children Act was to improve their position as litigants, and in the light of the implications of Article 6 of the Human Rights Act 1998 (rights to a fair trial), this is a worrying finding. As discussed in Chapter 4, some poor-quality letters of instruction from advocates on behalf of parents was only one part of the reason for rejecting these parties. Issues of professional prestige and reputation also determined consultants' practices. Accepting instructions on behalf of parents was not viewed as carrying much prestige. This finding requires wider discussion in both legal and clinical arenas.

Poor-quality instructions also emanated from some local authorities. This finding also requires discussion, especially in the light of subsequent proposals for improved collaboration between health and social services (see above). There are indications that there will have to be some very careful monitoring at a local level if any new collaborative arrangements are not to fall at the starting post because of continued poor instructing practices.

Second, wider discussion of the advantages and disadvantages of joint letters of instruction by child psychiatrists is necessary. The experiences of these consultants confirmed the findings of earlier national research during the mid-1990s: joint instructions tended to be a minority and sometimes controversial approach.[19] Practices are said to be changing following further directions from the Family Division (see Chapter 4, note 14) and most anecdotal evidence supports this. But further independent research is necessary to verify, for example, the magnitude of change and whether it has been successful in reducing the duration of public law cases. Existing evidence indicates it has not.

Third, these and other consultants[20] have identified some dangers regarding the use of joint letters of instruction – both in terms of the impact on the experts themselves and with regard to the likely impact on the profession and its role in litigation, where it seems their work may increasingly be unlikely to be subject to peer review. The child psychiatrists argued that, in the interests of children and the ethics of practice, work undertaken for the purposes of legal proceedings must be open to challenge and, if necessary, proceedings must allow for peer review.

This is *not* an argument for routine peer review of evidence but rather for recognition of the fact that expert knowledge is not a unitary

---

[19] In a national survey of 557 cases containing expert evidence and completed in 1994, some 6% were noted as containing a report or reports based on joint instructions (Brophy *et al*, 1999*b*, figure 4.1). In a court-based study undertaken in one local authority area during 1993/4 and involving 65 cases and 114 children, none of the expert reports filed were based on a joint instruction (Bates & Brophy, 1996).

[20] For example, Wolkind (1994, p. 1089) argued that, given that it is easy for individuals to develop and apply idiosyncratic sets of practices and viewpoints in this field, a major safeguard is for this work to be continuously exposed to peer review and audit in the same way as any other clinical activity in psychiatry.

category of knowledge – it is a dynamic and evolving body – and that experts are not infallible – nor do most wish to be seen as such. Indeed, it seems at times that some child psychiatrists are more concerned about issues of due process and getting it right for the child than some courts and policy makers in this field.

There is still much room for improvement in the way in which expert knowledge reaches the legal arena but reducing practices to what has been referred to as a 'one-shot lottery' may backfire. This is especially so if some child psychiatrists doubt the rationality and the ethics of a single expert in all cases and vote with their feet by removing their services – as some very experienced consultants did, on ethical grounds, when cuts resulted in the loss of their multi-disciplinary teams for this work in the early 1990s.

It is also important to keep the issue of peer review through the use of a second opinion in perspective. Contrary to received wisdom in this field, the research indicated that most cases involving expert evidence in care proceedings did not contain expert evidence filed by all three major parties, and even where expert evidence was filed by more than one party it was not necessarily conflicting (Hunt & Macleod, 1998, paras 12.10, 12.14, 12.15; Brophy *et al*, 1999*b*, figure 4.1). Moreover, even where there was a conflict of expert opinion, that, of itself, did not necessarily lead to a contested final hearing (Bates & Brophy, 1996, chapter 7). Even at the point at which concerns about this issue were probably at their highest (the mid-1990s), research did not support the view that there was a multiplicity of experts in most cases, all addressing the same or similar issues and concerns.

Moreover, while the lack of supply of experienced child psychiatrists clearly added to some delay in some cases, research demonstrated they were often not the only or even the major cause of delay.[21] However, at times, it appears that experts tended to become a somewhat convenient scapegoat in a system that was failing to achieve its initial objective of reducing the duration of care proceedings.

Thus, retaining effective avenues through which parties, if necessary, can obtain a second opinion is unlikely to open the floodgates. Moreover, retaining the *principle* of access to peer review of expert evidence in highly complex cases is a fundamental feature of social justice and thus viewed as an essential feature of proceedings by both guardians (Brophy & Bates, 1998) and experts themselves. It is also arguably underscored by Article 6 of the Human Rights Act – rights to a fair trial. The implementation of this Act in the UK in October 2000

---

[21] In a national sub-sample of 148 cases involving experts, guardians identified experts as the cause of delay in only 22% of cases (Brophy *et al*, 1999*b*, table 4.13).

makes it all the more important that careful attention is given to this issue both by courts and by experts.

### Setting a new clinical agenda

'Law' has clearly imposed a new agenda on the work of experts and, for the child psychiatrists in this study at least, one of the consequences of that exercise has been for some to begin rethinking the clinical agenda for this field of practice. As outlined under the heading 'Clinicians' responses to the new legal agenda' above, issues of ethics and practice are often highly interrelated. It appears that something of the spirit that originally underscored the Children Act 1989 – the principles of early inter-agency cooperation, the centrality of early support for children and parents, and the need to take a holistic approach – has led some consultants at least to consider that a new agenda is now necessary for their work in child protection litigation.

As indicated above, this agenda is not limited to a need to debate appropriate ethics for medico-legal assessments and views about separating assessment from treatment. It also covers such issues as the recording of treatment needs of children in court reports. As Chapter 3 demonstrates, consultants expressed dilemmas about where to pitch recommendations for future treatment – most positioned these somewhere between assessed needs and likely available clinical resources. But there was a strong argument for *both* categories of information appearing in reports. This is partly because courts should be given undiluted information on children's needs, and partly because health services should have an accurate source of data to help managers plan appropriate provision for this group of currently somewhat 'invisible' children. Formal recording of both sets of information may also help central government and local NHS trust managers and clinicians to reassess the low clinical priority that is frequently accorded to this group of children.[22]

As outlined in Chapter 5, the specialists in this study did not indicate substantial discomfort about dealing with the conceptual framework that 'law' is said to impose on their work (e.g. King & Trowell, 1992, p. 92), in relation to either the types of questions put to them by parties, or experiences under cross-examination in court. Most had no recent experience of being pressured to oversimplify their work or to make categorical statements in court. Indeed, consultants indicated that, with regard to the status of so-called soft (interpretive) evidence, they

---

[22] Subsequent amendments to care planning by local authorities also offer the potential for improvements in this field.

have made considerable progress in what was termed an educative exercise with both advocates and judges.

Equally, and *perhaps* surprisingly, experiences in the witness box have not resulted in considerable criticism of the adversarial nature of proceedings.[23] On the contrary, the consultants saw that as a necessary part of the exercise for both courts and clinicians in trying to get it right for children. Most consultants were emphatic: their evidence must be open to testing and, *if necessary*, subject to peer review. The possibility that this could happen was seen as important and helpful to clinicians when preparing their reports.

Finally, care proceedings under the Children Act were seen as a considerable improvement compared with previous proceedings; however, some of that progress was viewed as very fragile and indications were that there is little room for complacency. For example, the complaint by these consultants that case management is inconsistent because judges and magistrates do not generally reserve cases is not unique – it is shared by guardians and substantiated by research – and it does highlight complex problems for the organisation and admin- istration of family courts. There is ad hoc evidence that some courts do attempt to reserve highly complex cases, but this is by no means a national policy and for some courts it remains almost impossible. This judicial discontinuity was also found by Hunt & Macleod (1998, paras 9.14–16). These researchers reported that what was striking in their research in courts was that at no one level of court was continuity of tribunal achieved in more than a third of cases – and indeed two-fifths in the family proceedings courts and half in the High Court did not come before the same adjudicators twice. Like the consultants in this study, Hunt & Macleod argue that, to be effective, case management has to be seen as a continuous rather than episodic process.

Other practitioners and writers in this field (e.g. Ryan, 1994, p. 17) have pointed out that although the Children Act 1989 achieved some clarification and simplification of legislation and some undeniable

---

[23] Although one might have predicted that outcome from this sample since the consultants were selected only if still accepting instructions. Thus, it could be argued that this sample is likely to be less critical of proceedings than a randomised national sample, which would include people who no longer accepted instructions. Equally, as King & Trowell (1992, pp. 92–93) point out, this category of consultants may in fact be those who have developed strategies for survival in the legal arena. The point at which we part company from King & Piper's (1990) theoretical work in this field is the predetermined nature of the analysis offered. This study suggests that a much more interactive and multi-dimensional model is appropriate in understanding and theorising about the relationship between law and the 'psy' disciplines.

improvements to proceedings, it failed to introduce what has been termed 'a proper family court structure'. Although debate continues about this model, most are agreed that continuity of court tribunal and geographical location would assist many aspects of family proceedings.

However, as this study found, there are a number of questions for current proceedings that remain relevant whether or not that model is ultimately introduced. Broader questions need to be addressed about how principles of social justice can be furthered, particularly for parents, and about how adequate and independent testing of evidence could be improved. These principles of legal practice remain important in any quasi-inquisitorial model of dispute resolution in family law.

The clinicians in this study argued that their discipline and their expertise had much to offer but with certain provisos. One point was unequivocal: experts do not bring with them a unitary category of knowledge; nor do they consider that they should, and that is seen as an advantage that is important for courts, lawyers and policy makers to understand. Experts do not offer a panacea – they are an important part of the picture but not its solution; few, for example, would support a system that in effect is trial by expert. Second, these clinicians consider they offer a health-based service, yet in many ways it remains something of a hybrid. Nevertheless, important skills and expertise have been built up in the decade following the Children Act 1989 and these must be protected, assessed, enhanced and replenished.

Discussions about the use of experts – at least at the level of policy – are frequently dominated by criticisms and they (and not their contractual or institutional frameworks) have sometimes become scapegoats in discussions about delay and cost in child protection litigation. In that debate there is often little space for reflecting on some of the achievements of the past decade. These include:

(a) the contribution of the new threshold conditions – the 'significant harm' criteria – in moving proceedings towards more evidence-based practice;

(b) the drive to address and change aspects of court 'cultures' and to increase the courts' understanding of specialist knowledge and expertise;

(c) the success of directions hearings in providing a forum in which parties are now made accountable for their actions and evidence is timetabled;

(d) increased transparency throughout proceedings;

(e) increased specificity in instructions to, and the work of, experts;

(f) increased recognition of the importance of multi-disciplinary education and training for all professionals working in the family justice system.

These changes marked the *beginning* of an exercise in making child protection litigation a multi-disciplinary, evidence-based endeavour. But these policy endeavours have no 'natural' progressive momentum. Like the highly vulnerable children and parents they aim to serve, without time and investment, initiatives will be unlikely to flourish. Experiences in other jurisdictions (e.g. New Zealand) demonstrate that radical reforms in family proceedings become tarnished where there is lack of funding. This can result from a lack of investment in family courts, in specialist legal and welfare advocacy, in the Community Legal Service Fund (CLS) (what was Legal Aid) and lack of funding and training for independent expert witness services. Within that reframed policy context neither child welfare discourses nor 'law' are likely to determine its route. And in those circumstances, the 'system' may well fragment and, mirroring the responses of the abused child, turn in on itself, exhibiting guilt, responsibility, self-blame and low self-worth.

# Appendix

As stated in the Introduction, findings from parallel research in this field suggested a tendency for parties to draw on rather different 'pools' of experts in the field of child and family mental health. There was also anecdotal evidence that some specialists had preferences in terms of the parties from whom they wished to receive instructions. Thus one aim of the study was to elicit the views and experiences of experts in each of those 'pools' and explore these issues. Earlier research had highlighted a number of problems with many local CAMHS. A further aim therefore was to explore the status of court work within the overall workload of clinicians in this field.

In terms of the 'pools' of consultants from which we wished to select a sample, notions of 'national' and 'local' experts were utilised as part of the selection criteria. This terminology is also applied in the text when describing aspects of practice. It does *not* denote different levels of expertise in any clinical hierarchy. As Chapter 2 demonstrates, all respondents were consultants, and some had national and international reputations in their specialist field. Rather, the terms are employed to denote the geographical boundaries within which consultants accepted instructions.

## The sampling procedure

Respondent selection occurred in three stages. First, a national survey of guardians in England and Wales (Brophy *et al*, 1999*b*) provided details of the panels[1] providing assistance to guardians in the form of

---

[1] Guardians ad litem and reporting officers are currently located in panels administered by, but separate from, local authorities. At the time of the fieldwork there were 59 panels (54 in England, 5 in Wales). This administrative structure changed following the introduction of a unified court welfare service – the Child and Family Court Advice and Support Service (CAFCASS) – in 2001. This service, the responsibility of the Lord Chancellor's Department, is a non-departmental government body.

information on and lists of experts in the field of child psychiatry. Eighteen such panels were stratified according to size into three bands,[2] and within each band six panels were selected to achieve a good geographical spread across England and Wales. Letters were then written to the selected panel managers requesting access to their list in order to assist the study in locating a sample of consultants undertaking instructions in public law proceedings.

Second, data from the lists supplied by panels were entered into a computer package. Frequency counts showed the number of times a consultant's name occurred on the lists (i.e. doctor's name appearing on up to a maximum of seven panel lists). Where a consultant's name appeared on three or more panel lists, these consultants were classified as working on a national basis. In practice, the national list closely resembled a list of clinicians we had already compiled whose names occurred repeatedly in this field.[3] These psychiatrists were well known by reputation, and were often attached to major teaching hospitals or well-known institutions in the field of child and family health.

Consultants appearing on a maximum of two panels were classified as local experts (i.e. limiting their instructions in terms of close, usually neighbouring county boundaries). Six consultants were randomly selected from each of the three bands identified above (upper, middle and lower). Following selection, the institutional location of these consultants was checked to see if we had achieved a reasonably good geographical spread across England and Wales (i.e. consultants working in local services in the North East, the North West, the Midlands, East Anglia, the South East and South West, inner and outer London, the West Country and Mid and South Wales). The selected consultants were then contacted first by letter, then by telephone to check that they were continuing to accept instructions in public law proceedings.

In summary, a mixed sampling method was adopted. Eighteen panels were selected and stratified by size and geographical spread. From lists of child psychiatrists provided by each of these panels, experts were identified according to whether they worked nationally or locally, and respondents were then randomly selected from that list. These psychiatrists were then contacted and inclusion in the sample depended on whether they were continuing to undertake instructions. The sampling procedure was therefore purposive but, within that framework, experts were selected at random. While we cannot

---

[2] Panels banded by membership size: upper band, 124–26; middle band, 25–17; lower band, below 17.

[3] Identified in case law, commercial directories of experts, earlier studies within the same project and from publications in the field of child abuse/neglect.

generalise all the practices described here to all child psychiatrists instructed in proceedings, the procedure allowed for a range of experiences and views. The study thereby allows the generation of qualitative hypotheses with regard to a number of key issues surrounding the activities that consultants now undertake in care proceedings, and the contractual avenues through which their services are currently provided.

# References

Adcock, M. (1991) Significant harm: implications for the exercise of statutory responsibilities. In *Significant Harm* (eds M. Adcock, R. White & A. Hollows), pp. 11–28. Croydon: Significant Publications.

Advisory Board on Family Law, Children Act Sub-Committee (1999a) *Contact Between Children and Violent Parents: The Question of Parental Contact in Cases Where There Is Domestic Violence.* Consultation paper. London: Lord Chancellor's Department.

—— (1999b) *Report to the Lord Chancellor on the Question of Parental Contact in Cases Where There Is Domestic Violence.* London: Lord Chancellor's Department.

Aldgate, J. & Turnstill, J. (1996) *Implementing Section 17 of the Children Act 1989.* London: HMSO.

Allen, I. (1988) *Doctors and their Carers.* London: PSI.

Appelbaum, P. S. (1997) A theory of ethics for forensic psychiatry. *Journal of the American Academy of Psychiatry and the Law,* **25**, 233–247.

Association of Directors of Social Services & Royal College of Psychiatrists (1995/6) *Joint Statement on an Integrated Mental Health Service for Children and Adolescents.* London: Royal College of Psychiatrists.

Audit Commission (1994) *Seen But Not Heard: Co-ordinating Community Child Health and Social Services for Children.* Abingdon: Audit Commission Publications.

—— (1999) *Children in Mind: Child and Adolescent Mental Health Services.* Abingdon: Audit Commission Publications.

Bailey, J. (1995) Time for change in traditional practices? *British Medical Journal,* **310**, 788–790.

Bates, P. & Brophy, J. (1996) *The Appliance of Science? The Use of Experts in Child Court Proceedings: A Court-Based Study.* Research report for the Department of Health. Oxford: Centre for Family Law and Policy.

Bebbington, A. & Miles, J. (1989) The background of children who enter local authority care. *British Journal of Social Work,* **19**, 349–368.

Bentovim, A. (1990) Family violence. In *Principles and Practices of Forensic Psychiatry* (eds R. Bluglass & P. Bowden), pp. 543–561. London: Churchill Livingstone.

—— (1991a) Significant harm in context. In *Significant Harm* (eds M. Adcock, R. White & A. Hollows), pp. 29–60. Croydon: Significant Publications.

—— (1991b) What is significant harm? A clinical viewpoint. In *Proceedings of the Children Act 1989 Course.* Occasional paper no. 12. London: Royal College of Psychiatrists.

Betts, P. (1988) Small stature and physical signs of abuse. *Journal of Social Welfare Law,* **2**, 79–81.

Blom Cooper, L. (1988) The role of law and good practice. *Journal of Social Welfare Law,* **2**, 99–101.

Booth, M. (1996) *Avoiding Delay in Children Act Cases.* London: Lord Chancellor's Department.

BRITISH MEDICAL ASSOCIATION (BMA) (1996) *Fees for Part-Time Medical Services.* London: BMA.

BROPHY, J. (1992) New families: judicial decision making and children's welfare. *Canadian Journal of Women and the Law,* **5**, 484–497.

—— (2000*a*) 'Race' and ethnicity in public law proceedings. *Family Law,* **30**, 740–743.

—— (2000*b*) *Child Maltreatment and Cultural Diversity.* London: Nuffield Foundation.

—— & BATES, P. (1998) The position of parents using experts in care proceedings: a failure of 'partnership'? *Journal of Social Welfare and Family Law,* **20**, 23–48.

—— & —— (1999) *The Guardian ad Litem. Complex Cases and the Use of Experts Following the Children Act 1989.* Research series no. 3/99. London: Lord Chancellor's Department.

——, WALE, C. J. & BATES, P. (1997) *Training and Support in the Guardian ad Litem and Reporting Officers Service.* Research report. London: DoH, Welsh Office, TCRU (available from TCRU).

——, BATES, P., BROWN, L., *et al* (1999*a*) *Expert Evidence in Child Protection Litigation: Where Do We Go From Here?* London: Stationery Office.

——, WALE, C. J. & BATES, P. (1999*b*) *Myths and Practices: A National Survey of the Use of Experts in Child Care Proceedings.* London: BAAF.

BULL, R. (1992) Obtaining evidence expertly: the reliability of interviews with child witnesses. *Expert Evidence: The International Digest of Human Behavioral Sciences and the Law,* **1** (1, May), 5–12.

BURROWS, D. (1996) Care proceedings after *Re H. Solicitors Journal,* February, 94–95.

BUTLER-SLOSS, E. (2000) SFLA Conference: Presidential Address. *Family Law,* **30**, 230–233.

CARSON, D. (1988) Evidence of emotional abuse. *Journal of Social Welfare Law,* **2**, 77–78.

—— (1990) Reports to courts: a role in preventing decision error. *Journal of Social Welfare Law,* **3**, 151–163.

CHILD AND ADOLESCENT PSYCHIATRY SPECIALIST ADVISORY COMMITTEE (1999) *Advisory Paper on Specialist Training in Child and Adolescent Psychiatry.* London: Royal College of Psychiatrists.

CHILD NEUROLOGY SOCIETY, ETHICS AND PRACTICE COMMITTEE (1998) Child neurologist as expert witness: a report of the Ethics and Practice Committee of the Child Neurology Society. *Journal of Child Neurology,* **13**, 398–401.

CHILDREN ACT ADVISORY COMMITTEE (CAAC) (1991/2) *Annual Report.* London: Lord Chancellor's Department.

—— (1992/3) *Annual Report.* London: Lord Chancellor's Department.

—— (1993/4) *Annual Report.* London: Lord Chancellor's Department.

—— (1994/5) *Annual Report.* London: Lord Chancellor's Department.

—— (1995/6) *Annual Report.* London: Lord Chancellor's Department.

—— (1996/7) *Annual Report.* London: Lord Chancellor's Department.

—— (1997) *Handbook of Best Practice in Children Act Cases.* London: Lord Chancellor's Department.

CLAUSSEN, A. H. & CRITTENDEN, P. M. (1991) Physical and psychological maltreatment: relations among types of maltreatment. *Child Abuse and Neglect,* **15**, 5–18.

COOPER, A., HETHERINGTON, R., BARSTOW, K., *et al* (1995) *Positive Child Protection: A View From Abroad.* Lyme Regis: Russell House.

COYLE, G. (1985) *The Practitioner's View of the Role and Tasks of Guardians ad Litem and Reporting Officers.* Essex: Barnardo's Research and Development.

DAWES, R. M. (1994) *House of Cards: Psychology and Psychotherapy Built on Myth.* London: Free Press.

DENT, H. & FLIN, P. (eds) (1992) *Children as Witnesses.* Chichester: Wiley.

DEPARTMENT OF HEALTH (DoH) (1988) *Protecting Children: A Guide for Social Workers Undertaking a Comprehensive Assessment.* London: HMSO.

—— (1989) *The Care of Children: Principles and Practice in Regulations and Guidance.* London: HMSO.

—— (1991*a*) *The Children Act Guidance and Regulations, Vol. 1: Court Orders.* London: HMSO.

—— (1991*b*) *The Children Act Guidance and Regulations, Vol. 2: Family Support, Day Care and Educational Provisions for Young Children.* London: HMSO.

—— (1991*c*) *The Children Act Guidance and Regulations, Vol. 3: Family Placement.* London: HMSO.

—— (1991*d*) *Patterns and Outcomes in Child Placement: Messages from Current Research and Their Implications.* London: HMSO.

—— (1995) *The Challenge of Partnership in Child Protection: Practice Guide.* London: HMSO.

—— (1996) *Implementing National Standards: A Guide Through Quality Assurance for the Guardian Service.* London: DoH.

—— (2000) *The NHS Plan: A Plan for Investment, A Plan for Reform.* London: Stationery Office.

——, DEPARTMENT FOR EDUCATION AND EMPLOYMENT & HOME OFFICE (2000*a*) *Framework for the Assessment of Children in Need and their Families.* London: Stationery Office.

——, HOME OFFICE & DEPARTMENT FOR EDUCATION AND EMPLOYMENT (2000*b*) *Working Together to Safeguard Children: A Guide to Inter-agency Working to Safeguard and Promote the Welfare of Children.* London: Stationery Office.

——, COX, A. & BENTOVIM, A. (2000*c*) *The Family Assessment Pack of Questionnaires and Scales.* London: Stationery Office.

DEPARTMENT OF HEALTH AND SOCIAL SECURITY (DHSS) (1985) *Review of Child Care Law: Report to Ministers of an Interdepartmental Working Party.* London: HMSO.

—— (1988) *Report of the Inquiry into Child Abuse in Cleveland* (chair: Dame Elizabeth Butler-Sloss), cmnd 412. London: HMSO.

DIGBY, A. (1989) *British Welfare Policy.* London: Faber and Faber.

DOBSON, F. (1997) Looking inwards, looking outwards: dismantling the 'Berlin Wall' between health and social services. Paper presented at the Annual Conference of the NHS Confederation, Brighton, 25 June and quoted in Hiscock, J. & Pearson, M. (1999) *Social Policy and Administration*, **33**, 150–163.

EVANS, K. (1983) *Advocacy at the Bar.* London: Financial Training Press.

GIBSON, B. (1988) The courts' dilemma. *Journal of Social Welfare Law*, **2**, 104–106.

GOLOMBOK, S. & TASKER, F. (1991) Children raised by lesbian mothers: the empirical evidence. *Family Law*, May, 184–187.

HALLETT, C. (1996) From investigation to help. In *Child Protection: The Ttherapeutic Option* (eds D. Batty & D. Cullen), pp. 1–12. London: BAAF.

HESTER, M. & RADFORD, L. (1996) *Domestic Violence and Child Contact in England and Denmark.* Bristol: Policy Press.

HOBBS, C. J. & WYNNE, J. M. (1990) The sexually abused battered child. *Archives of Disease in Childhood*, **65**, 423–427.

HOPKINS, J. (1996) Social work through the looking glass. In *Social Theory, Social Change and Social Work* (ed. N. Parton), pp. 19–35. London: Routledge.

HOUSE OF COMMONS (1984) *Children in Care: Second Report from the Social Services Committee* (the Short report). London: HMSO.

HOUSE OF COMMONS HEALTH COMMITTEE (1997) *Fourth Report: Child and Adolescent Mental Health Services*, HC26-1. London: HMSO.

HUNT, J. (1993) *Local Authority Wardships Before the Children Act: The Baby or the Bath Water?* London: HMSO.

—— & MACLEOD, A. (1998) *Statutory Intervention in Child Protection: Thematic Summary.* Centre for Socio-Legal Studies, School for Policy Studies, University of Bristol.

—— & —— (1999) *The Best Laid Plans: Outcomes of Judicial Decisions in Care Protection Cases.* London: Stationery Office.

HYAM, M. (1992) *Advocacy Skills* (2nd edn). London: Blackstone.

JAMES, A. (1992) An open or shut case? Law as an autopoietic system. *Journal of Law and Society*, **19**, 272–283.

JAMES, D. S. (1995) Limitations of expert evidence: conference report. *Journal of the Royal College of Physicians of London*, **29**, 50–52.

JONES, D. P. H. (1991) *Working with the Children Act: Tasks and Responsibilities of the Child and Adolescent Psychiatrist*. Occasional paper no. 12. London: Royal College of Psychiatrists.

—— & ALEXANDER, H. (1987) Treating the abusive family within the family care system. In *The Battered Child* (eds R. Helfer & R. S. Kempe) (4th edn), pp. 339–359. Chicago: University of Chicago Press.

——, BENTOVIM, A., CAMERON, H., *et al* (1991) Significant harm in context: the child psychiatrist's contribution. In *Significant Harm* (eds M. Adcock, R. White & A. Hollows), pp. 115–136. Croydon: Significant Publications.

KAPLAN, C. A. & THOMPSON, A. C. (1995) Emotional abuse and expert evidence. *Family Law*, November, 628–631.

KEENAN, C. & WILLIAMS, C. (1993) Expert witness in child sexual abuse cases. *Medical Law International*, **1**, 57–71.

KING, M. (1981) Welfare and justice. In *Childhood, Welfare and Justice* (ed. M. King), pp. 105–134. London: Batsford.

—— (1990) Child welfare within law: the emergence of a hybrid discourse. *Journal of Law and Society*, **18**, 303–322.

—— (1991) Children and the legal process: views from a mental health clinic. *Journal of Social Welfare and Family Law*, **4**, 269–284.

—— & PIPER, C. (1990) *How the Law Thinks About Children*. Aldershot: Gower.

—— & TROWELL, J. (1992) *Children's Welfare and the Law: The Limits of Legal Intervention*. London: Sage.

LAU, A. (1991) Cultural and ethnic perspectives on significant harm: its assessment and treatment. In *Significant Harm* (eds M. Adcock, R. White & A. Hollows), pp. 101–114. Croydon: Significant Publications.

LAW COMMISSION (1986) *Review of Child Law: Custody*. Working paper no. 96. London: Law Commission.

—— (1987) *Care, Supervision and Interim Orders in Custody Proceedings*. Working paper no. 100. London: Law Commission.

LAW SOCIETY (1996) *The Directory of Expert Witnesses*. London: Law Society.

LLOYD-BOSTOCK, S. (1981) Does psychology have a practical contribution to make to law? In *Psychology in Legal Contexts: Applications and Limitations* (ed. S. Lloyd-Bostock), pp. xi–xix. Oxford: Basil Blackwell.

—— (1988) *Law in Practice: Applications of Psychology to Legal Decision Making*. London: BPS/Routledge.

LYNCH, M. (1991) Significant harm: the paediatric contribution. In *Significant Harm* (eds M. Adcock, R. White & A. Hollows), pp. 125–136. Croydon: Significant Publications.

LYON, C. (1988) From diagnosis to evidence: an examination of two cases illustrating problems of such a transition in situations involving potential emotional abuse of children. *Journal of Social Welfare Law*, **2**, 88–93.

MAITRA, B. (1995) Giving due consideration to the family's racial and cultural background. In *Assessment of Parenting: Psychiatric and Psychological Contributions* (eds P. Reder & C. Lucey), pp. 151–165. London: Routledge.

—— (1996) Child abuse: a universal 'diagnostic' category? The implication of culture in definition and assessment. *International Journal of Social Psychiatry*, **42**, 287–304.

MASSON, J. & MORTON, S. (1989) The use of wardship by local authorities. *Modern Law Review*, **52**, 762–789.

MILLHAM, S., BULLOCK, R., HOSIE, K. & HAAK, M. (1986) *Lost in Care: The Problems of Maintaining Links Between Children in Care and Their Families*. Aldershot: Gower.

MORRISON, T. (1991) Change, control and the legal framework. In *Significant Harm* (eds M. Adcock, R. White & A. Hollows), pp. 85–100. Croydon: Significant Publications.

MURFITT, R. (2000) Professional accountability of expert witnesses in the family court. *International Family Law*, September, 99–101.

NAPLEY, D. (1975) *The Techniques of Persuasion*. London: Sweet and Maxwell.

NEWHAM SOCIAL SERVICES (1999) *A Cry in the Dark: Children and Domestic Violence.* London: Newham Social Services/East Ham and The City Health Authority.

NHS EXECUTIVE, NORTH WEST REGIONAL OFFICE (1977) *Child and Adolescent Mental Health: A Review of Services in the North West.* Warrington: NHS Executive.

NHS HEALTH ADVISORY SERVICE (1995) *Child and Adolescent Mental Health Services: Together We Stand.* London: HMSO.

O'BRIEN, K. P. (1998) Pivotal issues in forensic psychiatry. *Australian and New Zealand Journal of Psychiatry,* **32**, 1–5.

OTWAY, O. (1996) Social work with children and families: from child welfare to child protection. In *Social Theory, Social Change and Social Work* (ed. N. Parton), pp. 152–171. London: Routledge.

PARTON, N. (1996) Social theory, social change and social work: an introduction. In *Social Theory, Social Change and Social Work,* (ed. N. Parton), pp. 4–18. London: Routledge.

PATTON, M. Q. (1990) *Qualitative Evaluation and Research Methods* (2nd edn). Newbury Park: Sage.

PLOTNIKOFF, J. & WOLFSON, R. (1994) *Timetabling of Interim Care Orders Study.* London: DoH/SSI.

RAPPEPORT, J. R. (1999) Thirty years and still growing. *Journal of the American Academy of Psychiatry and the Law,* **27**, 273–277.

RICHARDS, M. P. A. (1988) Developmental psychology and family law: a discussion paper. *British Journal of Developmental Psychology,* **6**, 169–182.

ROBERTS, R. E. I. (1994) The trials of an expert witness. *Journal of the Royal Society of Medicine,* **87**, 628–631.

ROBINSON, J. (1996) Social workers – investigators or enablers? In *Child Protection: The Therapeutic Option* (eds D. Batty & D. Cullen), pp. 30–37. London: BAAF.

ROYAL COLLEGE OF PSYCHIATRISTS' SPECIAL WORKING PARTY ON CLINICAL ASSESSMENT AND MANAGEMENT OF RISK (1996) *Assessment and Clinical Management of Risk of Harm to Other People.* Council report no. CR53. London: Royal College of Psychiatrists.

RYAN, M. (1994) *The Children Act 1987: Putting it into Practice.* Aldershot: Arena.

SACKETT, V. L., ROSENBERG, W. M. C., MUIR GRAY, J. A., *et al* (1996) Evidence based medicine: what it is and what it isn't. *British Medical Journal,* **312**, 71–72.

SAGATUN, I. J. (1991) Expert witnesses in child abuse cases. *Behavioral Sciences and the Law,* **9**, 201–215.

SEPPING, P. (1992) A future for children's mental health services. *Panel News – Independent Representation of Children In Need,* **5** (4), 23–25.

SIMON, R. I. & WETTSTEIN, R. M. (1997) Towards development of guidelines for the conduct of forensic psychiatric examinations. *Journal of the American Academy of Psychiatry and the Law,* **25**, 17–30.

SMITH, R. & WYNNE, B. (eds) (1989) *Expert Evidence: Interpreting Science in the Law.* London: Routledge.

SPICER, D. (1996) An injudicious approach to child protection. In *Child Protection: The Therapeutic Option* (eds D. Batty & D. Cullen), pp. 13–29. London: BAAF.

STURGE, C. (1992) Dealing with the courts and parenting breakdown. *Archives of Disease in Childhood,* **67**, 745–750.

THOBURN, J. (1994) *Child Placement: Principles and Practice* (2nd edn). Aldershot: Arena.

TROWELL, J. (1991) What is happening to mental health services for children and young people and families? *Association of Child Psychology and Psychiatry Review and Newsletter,* **13**(5), 12–15.

TUFNELL, G. (1993*a*) Psychiatric reports in child care cases: what constitutes 'good practice'? *Association of Child Psychology and Psychiatry Review and Newsletter,* **15**(5), 219–224.

—— (1993*b*) Judgements of Solomon: the relevance of a systems approach to psychiatric court reports in child care cases. *Journal of Family Therapy,* **15**, 413–432.

—— & SEYMOUR, C. (1993) Loss of multidisciplinary teams (letter to the Editor). *Association of Child Psychology and Psychiatry Review and Newsletter*, **15**, 159.

——, ——, ARNOLD, R., *et al* (1993) Child abuse and neglect: the development of a consultation workshop. *Association of Child Psychology and Psychiatry Review and Newsletter*, **15**(1), 7–14.

——, COTTRELL, D. & GEOGIADES, D. (1996) Good practice for expert witnesses. *Clinical Child Psychology and Psychiatry*, **1**, 365–383.

WALL, N. (1995) The judicial role in interdisciplinary co-operation. *Representing Children*, **8**(2), 52–55.

—— (2000) *Handbook for Expert Witnesses in Children Act Cases.* Bristol: Family Law.

WEBSTER, C. (1988) *The Health Service Since the War, Vol. 1: Problems of Health Care – The NHS Before 1957.* London: HMSO.

WHITE, R. (1991) Examining the threshold criteria. In *Significant Harm* (eds M. Adcock, R. White & A. Hollows), pp. 3–10. Croydon: Significant Publications.

—— (1993) The Children Act 1989 (letter to the Editors). *Association of Child Psychology and Psychiatry Review and Newsletter*, **15**(4), 203–204.

—— (1998) Significant harm: legal applications. In *Significant Harm: Its Management and Outcome* (2nd edn) (eds M. Adcock & R. White), pp. 9–32. Croydon: Significant Publications.

WOLKIND, S. (1988) Signs of emotional abuse. *Journal of Social Welfare Law*, **2**, 87–88.

—— (1993) The 1989 Children Act: a cynical view from an ivory tower (letter to the Editors). *Association of Child Psychology and Psychiatry Review and Newsletter*, **15**(1), 40–41.

—— (1994) Legal aspects of child care. In *Child and Adolescent Psychiatry: Modern Approaches* (3rd edn) (eds M. Rutter, E. Taylor & L. Hersov). London: Blackwell Scientific.

# Index

Coventry University